I Can See!

"I Can See!"

Can Surgery Get Rid of Your Glasses?

by

J. Luther Crabb, M.D.

an Osler House book

Peachtree Publishers, Ltd.

1988

Osler House
A Division of Peachtree Publishers, Ltd.
Memphis Office: 1407 Union Avenue
401 Mid Memphis Tower
Memphis TN 381838
Atlanta Office: 494 Armour Circle, N.E.
Atlanta, Georgia 30324

Now Lazier 2004 Surgery

Library of Congress Cataloging-in-publication Data

Crabb, J. Luther 1941-
I CAN SEE!
1. Keratotomy, Radial 1. Title
RE36.C73 1988 617.7-55 88-5124
(PBK)
ISBN-0-918518-70-9

Cover Design by Larry Pardue
Typography by Patterson Publications, Inc.

And they shall soar on wings like eagles.
Isaiah 40:31

ACKNOWLEDGMENTS

I would take advantage of the space I have been assigned here to make sure that the important people in my life are made aware that I realize their contributions to my work and the formation of my values.

First, my parents, Mr. and Mrs. O. H. Crabb, taught me that a man's worth cannot be measured by his possessions.

My sons, Jason and Alex, loaned me their computers and taught me how to use them to prepare this manuscript.

Samuel B. Johnson, M. D., was willing to see more than a gray-haired doctor when I applied for one of his prized ophthalmology residencies, and he made it possible for me to learn this magnificent art. This was the turning point in my life, as far as I can determine at this time.

My wife, Faye, has worked with me day in and day out, sharing the joys and sorrows of those afflicted with various eye diseases. She has seen me at my best and my worst, and she is still here. As long as I have her, I have enough.

And to my editor, Dr. Roger R. Easson, who helped me to transform ideas into language, thank you.

TABLE OF CONTENTS

LIST OF ILLUSTRATIONS

Figures

LIST OF ILLUSTRATIONS CONTINUED

Disclaimer

Radial Keratotomy is elective surgery. Knowledge about Radial Keratotomy is expanding rapidly. You should make your decision about whether or not to have this surgery only after consulting your physician for the most current information and for any factor that might affect your personal decision.

Do not decide whether or not to have Radial Keratotomy based solely on the information in this book.

I Can See!

1

The History of Radial Keratotomy

The attempt to correct Myopia surgically has three different origins. As with many other amazing contemporary inventions, this type of correction was first proposed by none other than the famed Renaissance Italian genius, Leonardo da Vinci, who wrote of such a possibility in his notebooks as he considered the anatomy of the eye and the mechanism of perception. Like so many of his inventions, this one lay forgotten as these wondrous notebooks were lost for hundreds of years, hidden and untouched on the dusty shelves of an European library.

The second time this procedure was proposed was in the early 1950's when a Japanese surgeon, Dr. Tutomu Sato, began to experiment with corneal incisions designed to flatten the corneal curve. Sato performed the experimental procedure with disastrous results. Nearly seventy percent of his patients went blind as a result of corneal clouding. He failed because at that time, ophthalmology did not fully appreciate the crucial role the inner layer of the cornea plays in main-

1

taining the cornea's transparency. It has now become general knowledge that unlike the rabbit cornea which can regenerate itself if injured, the human cornea can tolerate virtually no violation of its endothelial cell layer. Much of the willfulness of the negative press Radial Keratotomy, or "RK" for short, has received in contemporary media, may owe its impetus to the abysmal failure of Dr. Sato's surgery. [See Tutomu Satu, "Posterior Incision of Cornea," *American Journal of Ophthalmology*, 33 (1950), 943-8; Sato and others, " A New Surgical Approach to Myopia, *American Journal of Ophthalmology*, 34 (1953), 823-9; and also K. Aaiyama and others, "Problems Arising from Sato's Radial Keratotomy Procedure in Japan," *CLAO J*, 10 (1984), 179-64.]

One of the basic principles of scientific discovery popularly detailed by James Burke's *Connections* [Boston: Little, Brown and Company, 1978] is that many of the great discoveries are not always the result of the energetic application of a systematic and rational experimental program to investigate natural phenomena. Rather they very often result directly from the happy accident which takes place within the experience and curiosity of the scientist who is properly trained to comprehend the importance of that accident. Scientific revolutions are made of such stuff.

This is exactly the process by which RK was rediscovered for the third time in 1972. In that year a nearsighted Russian lad fighting with his friends was struck by a rock which shattered his eyeglasses into hundreds of tiny fragments. Some of the pieces of glass went into his eye, cutting the cornea and causing him great pain. As luck would have it, this particular patient was taken to the famous eye surgeon, Dr.

The History of Radial Keratotomy

Svyatoslav Fyodorov, Director of the Moscow Research Institute of Eye Microsurgery, to determine if his vision could be saved. When this young man arrived, Dr. Fyodorov was already a great man who had achieved fame in his country through his ability to implement his forward looking research in a land where medical progress often comes about with great deliberation and an equal amount of delay.

When Fyodorov examined the child, he saw that the glass fragments had cut the cornea in several places. Because the glass lens had broken symmetrically, the lacerations were rather evenly spaced around the pupil of the boy's eye. Indeed, although the wounds had extended deeply into the cornea, none of them penetrated through to the very last layer of the cornea and consequently the interior of the eye had not been damaged. Fyodorov elected not to suture the wounds, as the eye would heal just as well without them. Furthermore, he would thereby spare the lad the discomfort associated with this delicate procedure and the subsequent stitch irritation. As Fyodorov continued to follow the child's progress, he was amazed by what he came to regard as nothing less than a miracle. Not only did the boy recover completely from the accident, but subsequently it became clear that he had also recovered his vision perfectly. In fact, he no longer needed glasses to see clearly with that eye. A lesser surgeon might have chalked up the "miracle" to an "interesting but inexplicable event" soon to be forgotten in the pursuit of a busy career.

Not Dr. Fyodorov!

Fyodorov realized what had happened was probably replicable, and that it held untold promise for the surgical correction of myopia or nearsightedness, and the wholesale elimination of the need for glasses and contact lenses. Consequently, Fyodorov immediately set to work trying to replicate the effect in animal studies. The results of these experimental surgeries demonstrated that not only was the effect replicable, but also that as the wounds healed the cornea became flatter in a fairly predictable way. More to the point his research demonstrated that he could cause more or less flattening of the cornea by changing the length of the incisions.

By 1974 he was ready to begin human studies with this surgery. The results of these studies were successful beyond Fyodorov's wildest dreams and soon the

---

RADIAL KERATOTOMY IS A RELATIVELY NEW PROCEDURE DONE IN THE UNITED STATES ONLY SINCE 1978.

---

surgery was in great demand not only from his own countrymen, but also as Dr. Fyodorov's fame spread patients from beyond the Soviet Union began to seek him out.

Today the Russian use of RK is massive. At the Moscow Research Institute of Eye Microsurgery as many as one-hundred Radial Keratotomy surgeries are performed per day by a team of five eye specialists each performing a single step of the complex and automated operation. Consequently, every three minutes a patient leaves the operating room. The brilliance of Dr. Fyodorov's innovative-conveyer driven surgical theater has greatly improved the efficiency of the procedure. In keeping with his visionary program, Dr. Fyodorov recently observed that he hopes to per-

The History of Radial Keratotomy

fect a robot which will assume particular surgical functions in the near future!

Most Westerners who are used to more personalized medical care would very likely find Dr. Fyodorov's conveyer operated surgery—which has borrowed the technology of the mass production factory and applied it to a human product—particularly appalling. But that may well be more a function of our cultural inhibitions than of his.

The patient's progress through this automated surgery is nothing less than amazing. At the beginning of their fifteen minute processing through this mechanized surgery, patients are given sterile gowns and prepared for surgery. Each patient is guided to an operating table where the head is wrapped so that the eye to be treated is exposed, and thereafter anesthetized. The conveyor belt is designed so that the gurney bearing the patient may be placed on one side of the stainless-steel and glass doors which seal off the operating room. When the windows open, the gurney and its patient are engaged and eased gently along the conveyer into a predetermined position before each surgeon. A coordinator who manages the whole process speaks to each surgeon through headsets keeping the team apprised of both the medical condition of the patient and the procedure to be performed.

The American appearance of the operation was launched when Dr. Leo Bores, a successful and well known American surgeon left his large ophthalmology practice to study under Fyodorov. Dr. Bores performed the first Radial Keratotomy operation in the USA in 1978 and things have never been the same since. To date hundreds of thousands of Americans

I Can See!

have undergone this surgery and the potential of the operation to correct many visual handicaps seems to be limited only by an exceptionally strong bias against eye surgery which seems to be peculiar to our culture.

2

The Hazards of Being a Myope

Myopia: Origins of the Word

The word "Myopia" comes from the Greek myops meaning short-sighted. The Greek *myops* is itself derived from the Greek root words *"myein"* meaning *"to close"* and *"ops"* meaning "an eye," a combination which suggests the squinting and blinking condition characteristic of the behavior of the nearsighted person as he or she tries to bring a distant object into focus.

A relatively new word, "myope," meaning a person who can see things nearby but sees things far off poorly and its derivative "myopia," designating the condition of the myope, came into the language only as recently as 1693, where it was first used in a translation of *Blanchard's Physiological Dictionary*. Such words, derived as they were from Latin and Greek originals, flooded into the language during the Renaissance as scholars and scientists strove to develop the vocabulary in order to facilitate their native language's ability to sustain scientific discussions which characterized the technological revolution then

7

remaking the British intellectual landscape. Such so called "aureate" diction quickly replaced more ordinary English words in technical discussions.

The popular word in earlier periods for this condition was, however, something infinitely less flattering than "myopia." Ordinary people of the time called the condition simply "purblindness." The expression "pure blind" was in use as early as 1297 and meant simply "completely blind." It was used in this way many years later in Tudor England by no less a hand than the Bard of Avon himself, Shakespeare. Even in his day however it was increasingly rare in its use to describe someone utterly without the ability to see. The second meaning of the word "purblind" to designate someone we would today call "nearsighted" was in vogue by 1382, when it was used in this way in Wyclif's historic translation of the Bible. And it was used in this way in print until the latter half of the nineteenth century.

Myopia: A Visual Handicap

The fact remains, obscured though it may be by modern euphemisms, that the condition we call "myopia" or "nearsightedness" was for nearly four hundred years commonly considered a variety of blindness. Even the technology of ocular prosthesis such as eyeglasses and contact lenses has not completely eliminated the recognition that to be nearsighted is to be visually impaired and perceptually handicapped.

Next time you are in the bookstore or library count the number of people who are wearing glasses. Take that number and at least double it to account for those wearing contact lenses whom you may not recognize as

The Hazards of Being a Myope

"purblind." And you may begin to see the dimensions of the physical impairment for which we wear some kind of compensatory mechanical device. Of course, other kinds of visual impairment such as astigmatism or farsightedness may account for the use of such gear, but in contexts like the library or bookstore my bet would be that myopia is by far the most frequent problem these individuals exhibit. At least it pleases me to think that those of us who suffer from myopia are on the whole a more intelligent, and hence a more bookish, lot.

This book is about purblindness, or as we call it most often today, "nearsightedness." In particular, it is a book I have written for people who are handicapped by myopia and are considering the use of a new surgical technique called radial keratotomy to correct the defect. And as radial keratotomy is a kind of surgery my patients increasingly demand from me in my practice as an ophthalmologist, I thought it might be illuminating to them to have the opportunity to read a book about the subject of myopia and RK as they consider their use of the technique.

By way of preamble to more technical chapters, I want to share with you some of my thinking about this visual handicap and what I have come to believe is the reason more and more people are recognizing the need for this surgery.

The Trauma of Living with Myopia

Each of you who have selected to read this book have had some experience that has provided you with dramatic evidence you need to correct your visual impairment. Like you, I was also nearsighted and for

I Can See!

many years I endured the problems we have all suffered trying to live with glasses or contact lenses.

I remember when I was in high school it became apparent to me that the football coach, who was always prospecting the student body for likely candidates for his particular sporting requirements, had designs on me. Clearly my large frame was showing signs of brawn of a suitable character, and in my gym class I exhibited a knack for catching the football. I wasn't the fastest runner, but if I touched the ball, my steely grip made it all mine. Well, as you might imagine, this coach started after me with an excess of enthusiasm. But as I had no appetite for knocking heads with big bruisers benefiting from glandular disorders of one sort or another, I managed to hold him off until I achieved my full size during my senior year.

More confident of my physical prowess, I decided to give the sport a try. After a few months of practice, it became clear to both my coach and me that blocking and tackling were skills I could not master entirely, but when they decided to throw the ball to me, I could really excel. As the season approached, the coach-inspired visions of football scholarships seemed to assure me that I would be in great demand by colleges everywhere, and that my future was guaranteed.

I was soon to learn that for the nearsighted no stadium full of cheers could repair the need for good vision. Like other nearsighted kids of my generation, I wore glasses and for some reason the existence of plastic lenses was a piece of vital information some intelligent adult had neglected to provide me.

As the parents of nearsighted adolescent males know too well, glasses seem to exist in a state of constant disrepair. I was always breaking mine and consequently, I was very protective of my glasses, so much so that I kept them in my pocket most of the time. During my first game, the starting player at my position suddenly came out of the lineup, and the coach turned to me and yelled, "Luke!" It was time for me to go into the game. Just as I approached the man whom I was replacing, I got a good look at his face. All his front teeth were missing! If scrimmage could do that to the teeth, I was instantly struck by what might it do to my face, let alone my fragile glasses. As I was a substitute, my helmet had no faceguard and almost by reflex I took off my glasses and carefully deposited them with a teammate standing nearby before I galloped into war.

As expected, the quarterback called my play. I was to run as far as I could into the opposing team's territory, turn and catch up with the ball. Snap! went the play and I was off, like a shot. I ran until I thought it was an appropriate time to be looking for the ball and turned in the maneuver I had practiced all summer. To my horror, my field of vision contained not a hint of the ball anywhere. Moreover, I stood on an apparently empty though very noisy field where none of my teammates could be seen. What I had done so well during daylight hours was nearly impossible under the glaring stadium lights. It came to me then in a horrific flash that I wore glasses for a very good reason and this was one of those times that the reason was abundantly clear. Suddenly, out of the fog which usually concealed objects at some distance from me, I caught a glimpse of the pigskin hurtling toward me right on target. Unfortunately, a defender with better eyesight was there to bat it harmlessly out of my grasp.

As you may imagine the visions of college ball began to fade with some abruptness. My bubble had burst!

Later in the game my now less enthusiastic coach gave me another opportunity to see if I could salvage my potential, and I was quick to realize that without glasses I had to come up with some innovative compensation. So this time when they called my play, I shot down the field and didn't even look for the ball. Instead, I watched the player who was dogging my steps to block the pass. When he began to act strangely, I knew that the ball must be on the way. I just let him bat it again, and then swooped in to catch it before it hit the ground. Instantly, I was a hero! But while I reveled in my moment of celebrity, my success was tempered by the sure knowledge that such creative compensation wouldn't work all the time.

As I grew older and sought to find my chosen profession, I began to realize how limiting my visual handicap was. I began to be sensitized to how those of us who suffer from this perceptual impairment were locked out of many opportunities which the visually normal members of our society take for granted. On occasion, I would even hear someone use the word "myopic" to describe a decision or an attitude in a particularly derogatory way, as in "Don't you think that you're being pretty myopic about this?" So that the word itself came to characterize behavior that was shortsighted and thinking that was out of focus. To suffer from myopia seemed a double affliction, one of poor eyesight, and by a metaphorical extension, an affliction of the intellect as well. Finally, I began to notice how few successful politicians and high flying corporate executives wore glasses. I began to catalog the professions we were denied access to because of our purblindness. We cannot be jet jockeys because the military will not allow us to take flight training unless our uncorrected visual acuity is nearly 20/20. Consequently, we are more often passengers than pilots.

Most professional athletic opportunities are denied us as they require better than average vision to develop the competitive levels of performance such hand-eye (or eye—foot as the case may be) coordination activities require in the arena. How embarrassing it is to have a game stopped because a player has lost his contact lens, or as happens increasingly, when a player must leave the game and require a trainer's assistance when his or her soft contact slips back under the eyelid! Consequently, we myopes are more often spectators than participants.

Most police academies and para-military security forces require high levels of visual ability. They argue that the plight of a nearsighted police officer whose glasses are knocked off in a scuffle with a miscreant would be extreme. As the suspect flees, will the officer be delayed in the pursuit as he hunts for his glasses? Will his aim be impaired if he tries to fire a warning shot or to apply deadly force to a fleeing felon? Such prospects pose too high a liability for most police forces, so we nearsighted folk are usually reduced to being the protected rather than the protectors.

I am sure that if you consider your own life and the experiences that have forced watershed decisions upon you, you will come to realize how often myopia has been a significant factor in shaping your identity. It may have been so integral an element of who you believed yourself to be that you may not have considered it a determining factor. The fact of the matter is that nearsighted persons are often relegated to professions in which myopia is not a handicap. We find ourselves populating positions as librarians, teachers, or accountants, as artists, draftsmen, or computer programmers. We make great preachers or rabbis or priests. We flourish as desk jockeys, and as lab technicians glasses are sometimes required. Our world of gainful employment is often limited to that in which the encounter-of-the-close-kind dominates, if you will permit me a cinematic pun.

The Hazards and Disabilities Created by Wearing Glasses

The choice of a vocation is not the only area of our lives in which the handicap reduces the number of our choices. If we choose to correct this handicap with glasses, we will quickly find our visual impairment also restricts the use of our leisure time. As any individual who is more than mildly nearsighted will tell you, any water sport is a real challenge. Swimming, especially competitive swimming, for the nearsighted is nearly impossible. Our vision is so restricted that if we swim without our glasses we miss out on half the fun. Skin divers may sometimes buy expensive masks on which their lens prescription has been ground directly into the faceplate glass. But that is an imperfect solution at best. It is only with great difficulty that either snow skiing or water skiing may be undertaken by wearers of glasses.

The Hazards of Being a Myope

Looking straight ahead, an individual with normal vision possesses a field of vision of approximately 180 degrees. If you wear glasses your field of vision is reduced to about 100 degrees, greatly impairing your access to the critical information your peripheral vision provides. Consequently, you may not notice that car which has failed to halt at a four-way stop sign, a child who is about to enter the street chasing his ball, or the oncoming tennis ball which has just left your opponent's racquet. Merely turning your eyes won't help because you run out of glasses. Instead you must turn your head, which requires much more time than moving your eyes would. Similarly, if you wear contacts you will find that there are limits beyond which you cannot look sideways. The eyelids cause the contacts to dislocate or become uncomfortable. The degree of disability caused by these phenomena has not been adequately evaluated from a scientific point of view, but everyone who wears glasses has his own experience base which will illustrate the point to his own satisfaction.

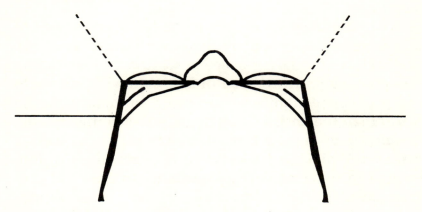

Figure 1: Wearing Glasses Limits the Field of Vision.

I Can See!

And how many fatal injuries have been caused because a myope was involved in a car accident, lost his
glasses, and when he extricated himself from the
wreckage wandered into the path of an oncoming car?
How many fatalities have lost their bearings simply
because they had taken off their glasses and in their
panic couldn't find them in time to escape a fire? All
of us who are myopes live with these paranoias every
day that our purblindness is not corrected. As the
posters say, "You are not a paranoid, if something is
really out to get you."

The constellation of irritants that wearing glasses
causes is as varied as each lifestyle. I hear my patients complain constantly about these small but constant irritations. One new mother complained that
she could not cuddle her baby while wearing glasses.
When a myope turns his head the whole field of vision
seems to move, and consequently he has to turn his
head farther than he might have had to normally,
hence the slight vertigo. And the sore bridge of the
nose; and the ears, the poor ears, especially of the
elderly.

The disability of myopia pervades every aspect of
our daily lives. When we work our lawns, we sweat
profusely and bending over causes the glasses to slip
off annoyingly. If we need them to see well enough to
operate the equipment necessary to manicure the
lawn, then the entire ritual of glasses cleaning, wiping
behind brow and ears must be completed before we
can continue. Repetitions of this ritual are often
enough to reduce a devoted gardener to a user of con-
tract lawn services. Sometimes we may resort to athletic eyeglass straps, but there is something about

sweat and glasses that no one loves for long.

How many times have I heard that people took their lives in their hands just to drive to my office to replace broken or lost glasses? And then there were the two weeks I spent touring Europe with broken glasses not seeing the Eiffel Tower, the Alps, and the Colosseum. Trivial? Perhaps. Unless you were that nearsighted individual.

The Cultural Implications for Myopes Who Wear Glasses

Each of us may have noticed the impact of our visual handicap upon our own lives, but have we noticed how intense that impact is upon those who would be elected to high public office, upon those who want to be the men and women in whom the public places its highest trust? Americans have a strong cultural bias against physical imperfection in candidates for high office. A visual handicap is only one of many imperfections which attracts the disapproval of the electorate. For example, does it strike you at all odd that only one bald man has ever been elected President since Grover Cleveland? That single exception was General Eisenhower, and he was running against another bald man, Adlai Stevenson. Shall we attribute to Gerald Ford's bald pate the responsibility for limiting a gifted politician to being the only appointed President who could not get elected on his own? As regards visual handicaps . . . of the fourteen Presidents elected in this century only the two Roosevelts and Truman were able to be victorious wearing specs. And had contacts or RK been as technologically advanced in their day they probably wouldn't have worn them either.

17

I Can See!

Teddy Roosevelt was such a vigorous man, and so personally popular that he could wear glasses and still win elections. Franklin Roosevelt's glasses were those odd pince-nez ornaments that he could remove quickly in public: he seemed always to have his glasses but not always to use them. Truman had the good luck to be Vice President when Roosevelt died in office. A wearer of glasses, he won reelection by only the narrowest of margins. Even so, he was known as the man no one loved, and his party denied him the right to run a second time. Those who know the inside scoop on the "Great Communicator," President Reagan, say that he wears one contact so he can read his teleprompter, and he is never caught wearing glasses in an official campaign portrait.

The Impact of Myopia upon Careers

The point of this small demonstration is that we are a culture obsessed with perfection. And if we are going to extend our trust in politics or in business we as members of this culture apparently would rather extend that trust to someone who is physically attractive and well dressed.

John Malloy's best-selling book Dress for Success has spawned a new industry of image consultants who are paid handsomely to consult with politicians, actors and actresses, and business executives to use their costumes to maximize their physical appearance in the wheelings and dealings of this nation's power elite. There are even individual fitness coaches who wheel their equipment-filled vans up to the homes of these high-rollers and give them personal fitness evaluations and workouts. More and more of these individuals are having facial plastic surgery to hide the ravages of their fast-paced, stress-filled lives. Weight-loss clinics, the notorious "fat farms," and the use of personal nutrition experts are a part of this new "physical perfection" industry which strives to provide the lean silhouettes thought most attractive by the power elite. Consequently, plastic surgery is no longer merely the province of middle aged women and accident victims. Today, plastic surgery is an option elected by more ordinary businessmen who wish to project as healthful and flawless a physical presence as possible. Indeed, it is fast becoming a clear necessity to those in corporate managerial ranks if they wish to maintain the competitive edge and hence to remain in the fast track of corporate advancement.

In this context, the use of eyeglasses falls in the same category as obesity, bags under the eyes, receding hairlines, and wearing last year's fashions; that is to say, they nearly qualify as a character defect. As I began to perform radial keratotomy I was amazed by the success stories my patients began to share with me on their follow-up visits. Indeed, when I had the operation myself, I saw my own income more than double as I laid aside my glasses. Should you think I am exaggerating to make a point, let me hasten to assure you, if you are a myope who wears glasses you may be suffering from career lag, though few will tell you that wearing glasses contributes to your inability to move forward as rapidly as you think you deserve. But one test you may resort to would be to observe those who are on the fast track to promotion, and see how many of them wear glasses, how many of them wear contacts, and how many are lucky enough to have normal vision.

I Can See!

Correcting Myopia With Glasses Affects Your Entire Ability to Perceive the World Around You

I remember when I was training to be an eye surgeon, I found it advantageous to remove my glasses while operating through the microscope. Most surgeons who wear glasses resort to this as it allows the focusing muscles of our eyes to rest while we are concentrating on the demanding manual tasks before us. To my surprise, I discovered that with my glasses off, I had to strain to hear what my instructor was telling me. It made me think I had learned to read lips as a result of my creative compensation for myopia.

> Radial Keratotomy is Not the Only Way to Correct Nearsightedness

Perhaps. But since we wear surgical masks during surgery that seemed hardly likely. More likely was the simple fact that without some correction of their handicap, myopes suffer a general deterioration of the "sensorium"—by which word we mean the total sensory envelope of stimulation provided by the brain as it processes and interprets its surroundings and creates our awareness and comprehension of the world around us. Moreover, this general sensory handicap cannot be easily explained to people who have normal vision.

Consequently, myopes have little choice. Until recently, we either had to suffer the indignities and nuisance levels of living with a mechanical assist of some sort or lose the ability to react to some of the stimuli which serve to enhance our performance. As

20

we shall see in later chapters, with the advent of RK this is no longer invariably necessary.

But glasses in all their delightful fashionable forms are not the only mechanical assist modern optical science has provided to correct nearsightedness. There is also the very considerable technological wonder of the contact lens.

The person who is generally given credit for dreaming up the idea that a glass lens could be worn on the eyeball itself is once more none other than that legendary Renaissance genius, Leonardo da Vinci. In 1508 he developed several ideas for changing the the surface of the cornea, a theory that was put in practice in the Eighteenth Century, when soldiers in the French Revolution disguised themselves by wearing glass shells that changed the color of their eyes.

The history of the evolution of contact lenses parallels the history of man's ability to shape transparent materials. According to one history of the technology of contact lenses, Eugene Fick, a Swiss physician, was the first in 1887 to grind down a small glass disk to wear on the eye and it was he who coined the term "contact lens." These lenses were a far cry from those in most common use today, as they were nearly as thick as the lenses of binoculars. One man was known to have worn these contacts for twenty years until his death in 1907, but fewer than two thousand people actually wore such contacts before the turn of the century. One of the most celebrated wearers of contact lenses was Madame Curie, who wore contacts laced with lead to protect her eyes from the radioactive materials she worked with after her discovery of radium in 1898. Few imitated her example, as they were heavy and dry. Throughout the first thirty years of this century, advances in grinding technology permitted the lenses to become increasingly smaller and lighter, but they were still heavy and difficult to wear. When plastics were discovered during the Second World War, technicians were quick to adapt the new materials in its many varieties to contact lenses. These new plastic lenses were hard and clear ; during the 1950's plastic contact lenses became the corrective eyewear of choice among the movie stars. But it was not until polymers were discovered in the 1960's that the amazing advances which brought soft contact lenses to the general public were possible.

Correcting Myopia with Contact Lenses

No technology which produces such marvelous advantages as those available with the new long-wear soft contact lenses is without parallel disadvantages. It should not be surprising, however, that given the obvious commercial impact of such news, these disadvantages are not as highly advertised as are the advantages.

Most contact lens wearers realize that for every hassle described above for wearers of glasses an equal trial awaits them. Contact lens wearers have not so much left off the nuisances associated with glasses as they have incurred an entire galaxy of new, if high tech, hazards associated with contacts. Of course, not everyone can wear these devices. Individuals who have severely dry eyes find it impossible to tolerate contact lenses. The natural tears provide the only source of oxygen which enables the external layer of corneal cells to survive. With a reduced flow of this vital liquid, wearing contacts is virtually impossible. [See Charles P. Adams, M.D. and others, "Corneal Ulcers in Patients with Cosmetic Extended Cosmetic Extended-Wear Contact Lenses," *American Journal of Ophthalmology,* 96:6 (December 1983), 705-9.]

Occasional Abrasions

The surface of the eye is a very delicate membrane, so that any artificial material which is in constant contact with it is going to cause some abrasion over time no matter how careful the wearer of a contact lens may be. Such abrasions heal readily when the lenses are left out of the eye for forty-eight hours. Such irritations are minor problems, though it means that a backup pair of eyeglasses must be in readiness.

Eye Infections

What is not generally recognized is that wearing contact lenses can cause severe eye infections, some of which can penetrate to the interior of the eye and destroy the whole organ in less than three days. Though rare, it takes only one instance to reduce an eye to utter blindness.[Louis A. Wilson, M.D., and others, "Pseudomonas Corneal Ulcers Associated with Soft Contact Lens Wear," *American Journal of Ophthalmology* 92:4 (October 1981), 546-54.]

Problems Caused by the Cleaning of Soft Contacts

The immensely popular soft contact lens must be treated very gently when cleaning. Unlike cleaning hard contacts, strong soap cleaners and heavy friction cannot be used to remove the protein buildup on the lens surface. A varied array of commercial products is available for such purposes. Some users develop an intolerance to the cleaning solutions owing to the presence of mercury-based preservatives used in the formula. This intolerance may cause redness and itching of the eyes, and when it is encountered it often causes the individual to discontinue wearing contacts altogether.

One additional feature adds a special kind of pain, a financial pain. In general, special enzymes are used to facilitate the removal of protein buildup. Some individuals are highly allergic to these enzymes which can trigger severe irritation. These enzymes can cause pitting of the contact lens surface. Such pitting can greatly reduce the life of the lens and by requiring more frequent replacement increase the expense of wearing them. [See Paul B. Donzis, M. D., "Microbial Contamination of Contact Lens Care Systems," *American Journal of Ophthalmology*, 104:4 (October 1987), 325-33]

Acanthamoeba Keratitis

One condition, acanthamoeba keratitis, is thought to be caused by contaminants in the solutions used to store the contacts when they are not in use. It occurs in highest frequency among those wearers who use salt tablets dissolved in distilled water for lens storage. Acanthamoeba Keratitis is very painful and can be blinding. Only rarely may the patient avoid corneal transplantation once this disease is established.

Giant Papillary Conjunctivitis

A significant percentage of soft lens wearers develop giant papillary conjunctivitis (GPC) which is manifested by the presence of visible bumps on the inner surface of the upper eyelids. The only way a cure of this condition may be effected is to cease the wearing of contacts entirely.

The Loss of Endothelial Cells

The most serious problem associated with the wearing of contact lenses is quite insidious. It is also quite predictable, and will affect everyone who uses these lenses for a significant period of time. Although this is critically important, it is very little publicized.

The cornea, which is only about one-half millimeter thick, is composed of several layers of cells. The interior layer is called the endothelial layer. These cells are so delicate that they are influenced by practically

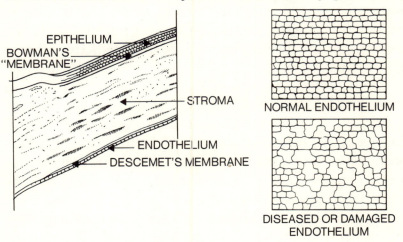

Figure 2: The Structure of the Cornea and Diagrams of Normal and Damaged Endothelial Layer.

anything which comes into contact with the eye. The endothelial layer is only one cell thick and its chief function is to pump water out of the cornea thereby maintaining the vital partial dehydration of the cornea which is necessary if it is to retain its transparency. Unfortunately in man these cells are totally incapable of replacing themselves: that is to say that when you are born, you have all of these cells you will ever have. When one of these cells dies, its neighbors widen and flatten to occupy its space, so that none of the interior corneal surface remains unlined.

There are several inherited diseases which cause a rapid loss of endothelial cells, worsening with advancing age, until the cornea becomes opacified, a condition which results in blindness. Corneal transplantation will help some of these conditions, but not all of them. A corneal transplant has a limited life in the presence of such diseases and is thus of little value if the patient is young.

Even in the absence of these diseases, there is an unavoidable attrition of the endothelial cells, so that all elderly persons have sustained significant loss of these cells. This is an important factor when eye surgery, especially cataract surgery, is contemplated as the surgery itself will destroy about ten percent of the endothelial layer.

Interestingly, what few advocates of contact wearers will tell you is that wearing soft contact lenses for ten years kills five percent of the endothelial cells. Wearing hard contact lenses for ten years kills ten percent of the cells. To place all of this into perspective, a donor cornea which is used as a transplant inevitably will begin its new life by losing fifty percent of these vital cells through the surgical manipulations which are part of the operation.

What then will happen to long-time wearers of contact lenses when they require cataract surgery? Many will need corneal transplants because to the natural attrition of these endothelial cells caused by the ageing process must be added the damage done both by the contact lens and the anticipated surgery. If the AIDS epidemic lives up to our expectations and our fears, it will most certainly limit the number of corneas acceptable for transplantation. That viruses can be transmitted by such transplants was dramatically demonstrated recently when a case of rabies was transplanted from the donor to the recipient with fatal results.

Certainly we do not know what the first generation of adults who wore contacts as youths will experience as senior citizens. Like so many new technologies we have not lived with contact lenses long enough to develop the kind of statistical studies necessary to make such predictions accurately. Is there going to be a dramatic increase of elderly individuals who go blind because they wore contacts when they were young? Clearly we don't know, but if I were a betting man I would lay odds on a dramatic increase in blindness among the elderly as these processes take their toll.

We may anticipate that people will continue to wear contact lenses for a long time to come. The manufacturers and the eyecare industry have a huge stake in maintaining this as the major form of treatment for myopia. How big is this industry? If twenty-three million people wear contact lenses, and each spends an average of one hundred dollars per year for lenses, cleansing solutions, and the high tech gizmos on the market to make care of such lenses easier, then we easily have an income of $2.3 billion for this industry. That's what you might call economic muscle of a major sort.

The size of this industry dwarfs that industry generated by radial keratotomy, the surgical correction of nearsightedness. Currently, the idea of eye surgery is very repulsive to young people, and this is a revulsion which the makers of contacts and eyeglasses have a vested interest in sustaining. As of this writing, fewer than one percent of all myopes in this country have chosen the surgical route to better vision. Yet I predict that within ten years, their numbers will become so great that contact lens and eyeglass wearers will constitute a minority among myopes. How can I be so optimistic? Simple. Because the surgery works. Because it is as safe as jet travel. Because the myopes who have the surgery are so happy that by simple word of mouth their joy in their liberation from contacts and glasses will convince others to have the surgery. Because many myopes will have to have the surgery simply as psychic self-preservation from the constant contact with those who revel in their new-found ability to see normally at long last.

3

The Anatomy and Problems of the Eye in General

A thorough knowledge of the contents of this chapter is not necessarily required in order to understand the principles of RK. However, I have found that the information contained in this chapter will serve to answer many of your questions and those of your family members regarding the need for this operation and regarding the problems of the eye in general. By no means is the discussion in this chapter meant to be more than the most general introduction to the anatomy of the eye and the problems most frequently encountered. For many of you this will be a review of some basic anatomy, for others it will provide a basis which will assist you in understanding the nature of radial keratotomy and its ability to correct nearsightedness. It is my hope that this chapter includes valuable groundwork which will allow us to discuss the potential of this procedure in your particular case with more clarity.

Some of the anatomical structures and related problems we will discuss in this chapter are as follows:

I Can See!

- Anatomy: The Muscles of the Eye
    - Associated Problems: Amblyopia
- Anatomy: The Cornea
    - Related Anatomical Structure: Endothelial Layer
- Anatomy: The Aqueous Humour
    - Related Anatomical Structure: The Ciliary Body
    - Associated Problem: Glaucoma
- Anatomy: The Iris
- Anatomy: The Pupil
- Anatomy: The Crystalline Lens
    - Related Anatomical Structure: Zonulae
    - Related Anatomical Function: Accommodation
    - Associated Problem: Cataract
- Anatomy: Vitreous Humour
- Anatomy: The Retina
    - Related Anatomical Structure: The Fovea
    - Associated Problem: Diabetes
    - Associated Problem: Retinal Detachment
    - Associated Problem: Color Blindness
    - Associated Problem: Night Blindness
    - Associated Problem: Retinitis Pigmentosa
- Anatomy: The Optic Nerve
    - Related Anatomical Structure: Optic Chiasm
    - Associated Problem: Multiple Sclerosis
- Anatomy: The Brain
    - Related Anatomical Structure: The Occipital Lobes

The Anatomy and Problems of the Eye in General

The Structure of the Eye

It is essential to understand the anatomy of the eye and its normal function before trying to delve into the abnormal states which represent disease.

The eye itself is roughly spherical in shape and has a diameter of about one inch. To our generation which so admires the miniaturization of electronic gear, especially the technology which has brought the computational power of the giant mainframe computers of the 50's and 60's into the generation of powerful laptop microcomputers of the 80's, the structure of the eye should be an amazement. The eye is the most complex sensory organ we possess and consists of nearly a thousand different parts supremely miniaturized beyond the wildest hopes of modern electronic technology.

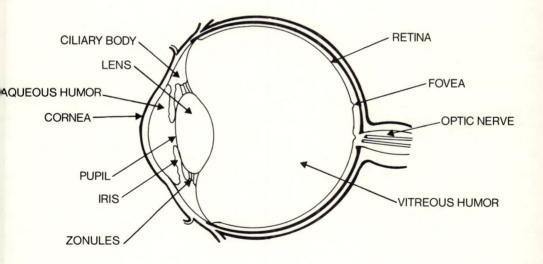

Figure 3: Detailed Diagram of the Eye.

I Can See!

The eye is so exquisitely sensitive that a normal person standing on top of a mountain in total darkness could see light emitted by a match struck fifty miles away.

Vision is the result of the complex interplay of the eye's receptors and that most fantastic of all computational structures—the human brain. Vision begins when the muscles of the eye coordinate the paired organs so that light reflected from the object of interest may pass through the cornea, the aqueous humour, the pupil of the iris, the crystalline lens, and the vitreous humour to strike the retina. In the retina of each eye, images are organized according to differences in contrast and color and transformed into electric stimuli which are transmitted through the optic nerves toward the two occipital lobes of the brain.

All parts of this system must be functional in order for useful vision to result, especially those structures found along the *visual axis*. We may imagine this axis as the imaginary line connecting the *fovea*—that area of the retina which is most packed with receptors—with the object external to the eye from which light has been reflected and upon which the eye is focused. When problems appear in this system, the difficulty of treatment is directly related to how far back into this system the disorder originates. The farther back, the more difficult the treatment.

Muscles of the Eye

There are six muscles attached to the outside of each eye. These muscles cause the visual axes of the two eyes to come to a point on the object which is the center of interest.

The Anatomy and Problems of the Eye in General

When this is impossible the patient will either see a double image or will learn to ignore the image seen by one of the eyes. If this condition is present in the first eight years of life, the child may be commonly described as having "crossed eyes" but, more technically, the condition is known as *amblyopia*. Patching the dominant eye will force the child to use the non-preferred eye, thus maintaining that eye's ability to see well. Alternative patching may be necessary to prevent amblyopia of the preferred eye. These measures are most successful if begun shortly after crossed eyes are discovered. A significant and permanent visual loss will occur if amblyopia is left untreated past the age of eight. After that time, patching may have less effect in increasing the usefulness of the eye.

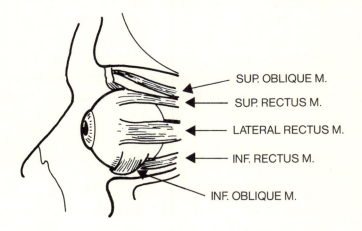

SUP. OBLIQUE M.

SUP. RECTUS M.

LATERAL RECTUS M.

INF. RECTUS M.

INF. OBLIQUE M.

Figure 4: The Muscles of the Eye and Their Attachments.

I Can See!

Not all children with crossed eyes will develop amblyopia, as some learn to use one eye at a time, alternating frequently between the two eyes. If their eyes are straightened surgically, they will continue to alternate, but the binocular vision necessary for development of good depth perception will not occur. Still, these individuals are able to function very well in our society.

The Cornea

The cornea, which is only about one-half millimeter thick, is composed of several layers of cells. The interior layer is called the "endothelial layer." This layer is so delicate that it is influenced by practically anything that comes into contact with the eye. The endothelial layer is only one cell thick. Its chief function is to pump water out of the cornea, thereby maintaining the vital partial dehydration of the cornea which is necessary if it is to retain its transparency. Unfortunately, in man these cells are totally incapable of replicating themselves: that is to say when you are born you have all the cells you will ever have. When one of these cells dies, its neighbors widen and flatten to occupy its space, so that none of the interior cornea remains unlined.

The cornea is one of the few tissues of the body which has no blood supply and derives all its nourishment from the aqueous humour and the tear film. It is the job of the cornea to bend the light that passes through it so that it will converge into an image by the time it reaches the retina at the back of the eye. The power of the cornea is usually insufficient to achieve this alone, therefore a second refractive medium, the crystalline lens, further contributes to this bending of the light.

The Aqueous Humour

The aqueous humour is a clear liquid continually secreted and absorbed which is produced by a portion of the ciliary body so that it is renewed regularly about every four hours. Its function is mainly to maintain the eye in a constant state of roundness and provide nourishment to the cornea and lens.

Glaucoma is the name given to a number of disorders in which eye structures are damaged by an imbalance in the production and removal of aqueous humour. Some glaucomas are slow and insidious. Others are acute and painful. All can cause total and permanent blindness. Unfortunately, like hypertension, glaucoma usually has no symptoms until great and irreversible damage has occurred. The only means of early detection is by an eye examination which includes a measurement of intraocular pressure.

The Iris

Beneath the aqueous humour is a delicate structure called the iris. This is the pigmented portion of the eye and is found in a wide range of colors. Though it does not matter what color the iris may be, eyes lacking color in the iris, such as in cases of albinism, are greatly handicapped. The pigmentation of the iris exists to block light so that it may effectively operate as an aperture for the lens.

The iris serves to regulate the amount of light entering the eye. When intense illumination is present,

I Can See!

the iris contracts its circular muscles to cause the pupil to become smaller, thus protecting the retina from undue exposure to potentially harmful levels of light. In darkness, these same muscles relax, allowing the pupil to enlarge, affording more exposure to the limited amount of light available.

The iris is controlled by involuntary smooth muscles operated by the autonomic nervous system. As a consequence of this, the pupil may be affected by the emotional state so that it increases in size with emotional arousal.

The Pupil

Oddly enough, the pupil is a non structure as it is the hole or aperture formed by the iris and through which the iris permits light to strike the lens and continue on to the retina.

Many disorders of the pupil can be traced to the brain and its emergent nerves, but some occur at the level of the iris itself. Unequal pupils may, or may not, be an important sign of severe disease in other parts of the body; thus, an eye examination is necessary to determine whether other tests are necessary.

The Crystalline Lens

The crystalline lens is a special structure which continues to bend light passing through the eye so that it is focused onto the retina. The process by which this is accomplished is called accommodation. Unlike the hard lens of a camera, to which the crystalline lens is often compared, the crystalline lens can change its shape to allow greater bending of the light waves when necessary. The radius of the lens is reduced for near vision, creating a more powerful bending of the light waves when necessary. Internal eye muscles act to cause the lens to become more round and more powerful during this process of accommodation, without which reading would be difficult.

The crystalline lens is built up of thin layers like a hailstone or onion, and is suspended like a hammock by fibers called the zonulae. These layers are built up during life as we continually add layers of cells to the lens. As we grow older, though this process slows down, more layers of cells grow onto the lens surface, gradually restricting the ability of the cells at the center of the lens to gain access to oxygen and nourishment. As these cells die, they harden, causing the lens to stiffen and limiting its ability to accommodate. At about the age forty-five the individual may begin to notice that small print is difficult to read even at arm's length, which is a symptom of a condition known as presbyopia. Reading glasses are generally prescribed for this condition.

The principle disorder of the lens is called a cataract, which occurs when the lens has lost its clarity. A tiny cataract can markedly reduce vision if it is located along the visual axis. Cataracts can be caused by trauma as well as a variety of metabolic disorders. Usually, however, cataracts are a product of the ageing process. The constant exposure of the lens to light gradually alters the chemical structure which is so crucial to the exquisite clarity necessary for good vision. It may be safely said that all persons older than sixty-five years have some degree of cataract. The mere presence of cataract does not mean that surgery is required, however. Each individual must decide

I Can See!

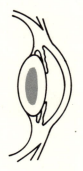

Figure 5: Diagram of the Eye with a Cataractrous Lens.

when visual function has been unacceptably reduced to such degree that he or she is willing to undergo cataract removal.

No medical treatment is available for cataract, although intensive research is underway in this area. Cataract surgery is not without risk, but over ninety percent of cataract operations performed are successful. New and highly sophisticated instruments have brought about a high rate of visual restoration for this otherwise blinding condition.

Vitreous Humour

The vitreous humour is a semifluid substance lying between the lens and the retina. It helps to maintain the shape of the eye, but it may be removed surgically and replaced with salt water without causing blindness. The vitreous humour is very important during the embryonic development of the eye, but afterward it may become a burden for two reasons. First, it is so thick that a hemorrhage occurring within the eye may

38

permit the blood to become entrapped in the visual axis and remain undissolved for months or years. Second, it is attached to the retina and can cause the retina to detach from the back of the eye.

The Retina

A thin sheet of highly specialized nerve cells covering two-thirds of the posterior surface of the eye, the retina is actually a portion of the brain which has budded out during gestation to form part of the eye. The word "retina" literally means "net" or "cobweb tunic" referring to the net of blood vessels which lies near the surface of the retina.

Oddly, the receptors which receive the light and translate it into the kind of electrical activity the brain requires do not lie on the surface of the retina, as you might expect. They lie on the back of the retina requiring that light first pass through the web of nerve fibers and blood vessels, in addition to three layers of supporting cells in order to reach these receptors.

Optically, then, the eye is wrongside out, a situation which is the direct result of the retina developing embryonically from the surface of the brain. The situation works, because nerve fibers avoid the central part of the retina, the fovea, where the receptors are packed exceedingly close together. Two kinds of receptors exist and are termed by their shapes, rods and cones. The cones function in conditions of high illumination and provide the necessary information for color vision, while the rods function under conditions of lower illumination and provide the necessary information for variations of gray.

R. L. Gregory, writing about these photo receptors,

observes: "It is worth trying to imagine the size of the receptors. The smallest is one micron, only about two wave lengths of light in size. The number of cones is about the same as the population of Greater New York. If the whole population of the United States were made to stand on a postage stamp, they would represent the rods of a single retina."
[See Gregory's extraordinary book, *Eye and Brain: The Psychology of Seeing,* third edition, revised, New York: McGraw-Hill, 1977, p.63.]

Damage to the Retina Caused by Diabetes

The retina has two blood supplies which are separate from each other and have virtually no overlap. If any part of this vascular system malfunctions, the whole visual process may be arrested. One of the most common sources of interruption to this blood supply is diabetes mellitus, which damages the retinal blood vessels, causing oxygen starvation in the retinal cells. The small vessels attempt to multiply to increase the oxygen supply, but these new vessels are inferior and often hemorrhage. This release of blood into the vitreous humour mechanically blocks vision and is but one of the many ways diabetes can cause retinal damage. It is important because it can be treated with lasers which work by creating heat that destroys tiny areas of the retina. The need for oxygen is thus decreased, and the new vessels will regress to a varying extent. It is ironic that to save the retina, we must sometimes destroy part of it.

Retinal Detachment

A number of mechanisms may cause the retina to become detached from the rear wall of the eye. This process of detachment usually begins with the appearance of a small hole in the retina. The semifluid vitreous humour may exert traction on the edges of this perforation, gradually causing the area surrounding the hole to separate from its supporting structure. Several degenerative disorders allow such holes to develop. For example, high myopia stretches the retina because the eye becomes larger than the retina can easily cover in this condition.

Spontaneous detachment may occur or mild trauma can trigger the event. Surgical treatment consists of bringing the retina closer to the wall of the eye where it was, then freezing the area, depending upon the resultant inflammation to create an adhesion between the retina and the outer eye wall structures.

Because early detection is the key to minimizing the damage caused by retinal detachments, if you experience what some patients have called "lightning flashes"—which are very bright, colorful, and continually repeated—you should see an ophthalmologist. If enough damage occurs to the retina, it does not matter how perfect the rest of the eye may be, vision will be lost.

Color Blindness and Night Blindness

Color blindness results from a malfunction of one or more types of the retinal cone cells, the specialized photoreceptors which function in moderate to strong illumination. The other type of photoreceptor, the rod cell, is responsible for vision in dim light, allowing us to find our seats at the movie theater after the picture has started, for example. Night blindness is one of the signs of retinitis pigmentosa, a potentially blinding disease which is usually inherited. There are many individuals who cannot see well enough to drive safely at night and who have no retinal disease. For these usually fair-skinned and nearsighted individuals, stronger eyeglasses may provide adequate relief.

The Optic Nerve

The optic nerve is a collection of the electrical transmitters of the retina which connect with the brain. The optic nerves from the two eyes join at a cross point called the optic chiasm and divide so that half the transmitters from each eye cross toward the opposite lobe of the brain where they penetrate to the visual cortex located at the back of the brain. This division brings the transmitters from the half of the retina nearest the nose in one eye, and merges them with the transmitters from the half of the retina nearest the temple in the other eye. In this way the optic chiasma enables the retinal transmitters to bring two views of the same part of the visual world together within the bilaterally symmetrical brain.

Many diseases can attack the optic nerve, but probably the most common is multiple sclerosis. In this condition, part of the covering of the nerve is destroyed, leaving the nerve less able to transmit its information to the brain. Color perception may be impaired in a way which affects the degree of contrast or saturation rather than the confusion of one color with another.

In addition, the optic nerve may be severely compromised by glaucoma. This damage seems to work slowly by initially wiping out peripheral vision and in later stages by compromising the central portion of the retina. It is very possible to have a patient who has 20/20 vision, but with glaucoma so severe that no peripheral vision is present. Such a condition would be like constantly looking down a long tunnel in the darkness. Although a person in this condition may see an object well, he cannot find it unless it accidentally falls along his visual axis.

The Brain

It is important to remember that the brain is divided into two halves of lobes connected only by one large trunk of nerves called the corpus callosum. Much has been written about the interworkings of this paired structure in the fabrication of consciousness. The nature of perception, and the way in which our brain is able to comprehend the world around us as a result of the sensory input of its senses, has been increasingly at the center of a major revolution in psychology and psychiatry during the last twenty years. [See for example, Robert Ornstein, *The Psychology of Consciousness*, New York: Harcourt Brace Jovanovich, Second Edition, 1977 and Judith Cooper and Dick Teresi, *The Three Pound Universe: The Brain,* New York: Dell, 1986.]

In general, it may be said that the brain is a highly integrated computational system which receives thousands of signals from its sensory organs as they interact with the environment. The speed with which the brain interprets these signals is much faster than the processing speeds of our fastest supercomputer and within nanoseconds the brain fashions responses to them. To understand the computational speed with which the brain responds to these signals, we need to

I Can See!

understand that one nanosecond relates to one second in the way that one second relates to thirty years. Most of these signals which the sensory organs transmit to the brain come from the eye, and six of the twelve cranial nerves serve the eye.

Most of this information from the eyes reaches the most posterior portion of the brain, the occipital lobes. Damage to this area can cause blindness, even when both eyes are perfectly normal. Most of the diseases of the brain involve strokes or tumors, or result from blows to the head. Many other diseases may be inherited, or may arise from some form of degeneration or infection. Any of these may affect the vision in one way or another. My point here is that any abnormal symptom of the eye should be investigated promptly because it may represent any of these brain disorders and many of these can be greatly alleviated or even cured by timely treatment.

4

Is Radial Keratotomy Safe?

In this chapter, I want to undertake an explanation of the risks involved with radial keratotomy, so that you and your family might be able to make an informed decision about the nature of this procedure and be fully aware of both the risks and benefits of this remarkable surgical correction for nearsightedness.

> THE RESULTS OF ANY SURGICAL PROCEDURE CAN NEVER BE GUARANTEED.

No surgeon can ever guarantee his work. Your eye surgeon will try to do everything within his power to minimize the risks of this surgery. His efforts to minimize your risk begin with a careful evaluation of the physical condition of your eyes, an assessment of the nature of your visual impairment and whether you will benefit from RK. Together you and your eye surgeon will consider the value of RK to your particular

I Can See!

visual circumstances and what tradeoffs you will make if you do or do not choose to have the surgery. Obviously, not everyone who comes in for an evaluation will benefit from the procedure. For some patients the operation would be inadvisable; for others their problem might be more successfully resolved with another kind of treatment program. After performing more than 2000 of these procedures, I have had a few patients who have had some annoying problem for two or three weeks following the operation. On two occasions a patient developed a sensitivity to light which lasted three or four months. Some of my patients, who had nearsightedness of such magnitude that RK could not fully correct it, still wear glasses, though these glasses have much thinner lenses than before.

> RK SURGERY IS SUBJECT TO RISKS ASSOCIATED WITH OTHER TYPES OF SURGERY.

In this chapter I would like to deal with a series of risks most feared as a result of RK. Some of these risks are real, many are not. So let us deal with each of them in turn as follows:

- The Risk of Infection
- The Risk of Weakened Eye Structure
- The Risk of Overcorrection
- The Risk of Unpredictable Results with RK
- The Risk of Cataract Formation as a Result of RK
- The Risk of Losing the Protection of Glasses
- The Risk of Corneal Scarring Caused by RK
- The Risk of Retinal Detachment
- The Risk of Losing Visual Acuity

46

Is Radial Keratotomy Safe?

The Risk of Infection

One of the risks of any surgery is postoperative infection. I know of one case in which the loss of an eye resulted from postoperative infection. The eye developed an infection which spread to the inside of the organ, and the doctor was unable to stop the bacterial growth until it had rendered the eye useless. The history of surgery over the last century has been a history in which the advances in understanding of the causes of infection and medicine's ability to combat the sources of such infection has been a major success story. The acceptance of sterile procedure and the discovery of antibiotics have been the two landmark developments in this success.

IT IS IMPOSSIBLE TO NAME ALL THE POSSIBLE COMPLICATIONS ASSOCIATED WITH RK AS WITH ANY SURGERY. THIS BOOK INCLUDES MOST OF THE COMPLICATIONS THAT ARE KNOWN TO HAVE HAPPENED OR THOUGHT TO BE CAPABLE OF HAPPENING.

In the case of RK, the cornea receives a series of very intricate incisions which remain open for about two days. After this period, the healing process will protect the incisions with a restored barrier to infection. During the two days prior to the surgery and the four days following the surgery, I prescribe the use of a specific kind of eyedrop—Tobrex®—which is a preparation of tobramycin. Theoretically, the use of Tobrex® prior to surgery will decrease the amount of bacte-

47

ria in the eye at the time of surgery, thus giving it a head start in the healing process. Although there have been no clinical studies which confirm the advantage of such practice, I have had good results with this procedure. And as they say in the military: "If it isn't broken, don't fix it".

During this window of vulnerability the most dangerous source of infection is the bacteria known as "pseudomonas." This bacteria lives in the very air we breathe so it is very difficult if not impossible to avoid it completely. However, the small amounts of pseudomonas found in the air are rarely sufficient to establish an eye infection; but, as chlorinated swimming pools and hot tubs are a notorious breeding area for pseudomonas, I make certain that all my RK patients know to avoid these areas completely for at least ten days following the surgery. [See Beverly J. Kush MS, and A. S. Hoadley, Ph.D. MPH, "A Preliminary Survey of the Association of *Pseudomonas aeruginosa* with Commercial Whirlpool Bath Waters," *American Journal of Public Health*, 70:30 (March 1980), 279-81.] The use of Tobrex® has proven sufficient to protect the eye after surgery provided that swimming and hot tubs are avoided. As a result of these and other precautions—as well as good luck—none of my patients has ever had an eye infection caused by RK.

The Risk of Weakened Eye Structure, or the Case of the Exploding Pig Eyes

When I first learned that this surgery was being done, I remember my initial fear was that the surgery would so weaken the eye that the patients would incur a tremendous risk of suffering an exploded eye if their eyes experienced any significant impact. Images of the aftermath of auto accidents or sports-related injuries for RK patients with apparently weakened eye structures plagued me. What active individual would want to risk a random encounter with a racketball, tennis ball, or an opponent's elbow in a pick-up basketball game after having had RK?

I attended a symposium in 1982 during which a presentation was made by a researcher which seemed to demonstrate that the eye would be fatally weakened by RK. In his studies RK-like incisions were made on the removed eyes of freshly slaughtered pigs. Then steel balls were dropped on the incised pig eyes from a variety of heights to determine just how high one would have to elevate the steel ball before the eyes would burst with predictable frequency. As a control group, pig eyes without RK-like incisions were also subject to similar stress and it was determined that a significant difference existed. The pig eyes with the RK incisions were weaker. The conclusion seemed inescapable. A patient on whom RK had been performed would seemingly have to endure an intolerably high risk of catastrophic injury from impact on the eye with a blunt object. [See also B. C. Larson, M.D. and others, "Quantitated Trauma Following Radial Keratotomy in Rabbits," *Ophthalmology*, 6: 90 (June 1983), 660.]

As a consequence of this evidence, for a period of at least two years, I put the idea of performing this surgery on my patients on the shelf marked "highly implausible." It simply seemed not to be in the best interest of anyone to have this procedure replace the use of contacts or eyeglasses. Meanwhile, no record of

I Can See!

an RK-weakened exploding eye appeared in the published literature. As time went on, I began to encounter in the medical literature reports of RK patients who had suffered injury as a result of being struck in the face with great force by blunt objects. [See for example, L. Spivack, M. D., "Radial Keratotomy Incisions Remain Intact Despite Facial Trauma From Plane Crash (Case Report)," *Journal of Refractive Surgery*, 3:2 (1987), 59-60.] The eyes were often injured, but the damage was internal and not related to any weakening of the eye resulting from RK. This evidence seemed to be in conflict with the studies performed on pig eyes until it was realized that the pig eyes had never had an opportunity to heal prior to being stressed. It would seem therefore that we had another of those proverbial instances of comparing apples to oranges.

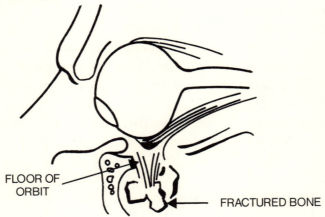

FLOOR OF
ORBIT

FRACTURED BONE

Figure 6: A Blow-out Fracture Is One Possible Result of A Blunt Trauma.

Is Radial Keratotomy Safe?

But let us be more technical, if you like.

When the eye suffers blunt trauma, we may say that in general two forms of severe injury are possible and one or the other usually prevails.

First the sudden compression of the eye transmits force to the orbit of the eye (bones, usually called the "eye socket") causing a fracture. Sometimes the eye must be lifted back up through the fractured bones immediately beneath the eye. Such a fracture is called a blowout fracture. Second, and far more commonly, blunt trauma to the eye results in the tearing of small blood vessels within the eye causing hemorrhages on the inside of the eye and immediate decrease of vision. If no critical structures are damaged, in most of these cases, the eye will regain vision in a few days, although there may be serious complications later. In neither of these two major forms of traumatic injury does the eye explode, except with some rarity, and then it is usually the posterior eye which gives way.

It is important to consider that RK works particularly because the incisions do weaken the cornea of the eye briefly. When the incisions are made the internal pressure of the eye causes the shape of the cornea to change to a more flattened central curve. By the end of three weeks, eyes corrected as a result of RK regain about seventy to ninety percent of their former strength. Fortunately, nature has provided us with at least three times the structural strength required so that three weeks after RK we can be relatively assured that the eye is not fatally weakened. During this period I caution my patients not to dive, to jog, to provoke their friends, or to engage in any activity which might cause a fall or a blow to the eye.

I Can See!

The Risk of Overcorrection

A very significant risk of RK surgery, and one which each prospective patient of RK must consider, is the possibility of overcorrection.

Overcorrection may cause the patient to be farsighted. Farsighted individuals must wear glasses to enable them to see for tasks near at hand as well as the observation of things at a distance.

IT IS POSSIBLE FOR VISION TO BE OVER-CORRECTED, MAKING IT NECESSARY TO WEAR OPTICAL CORRECTION FOR BOTH NEAR AND FAR VISION

"Farsightedness" is an unfortunate euphemism for this condition, as it seems to imply that the individuals who suffer this disability can see clearly at a distance. This may be true if the patient is a child, but as he or she grows older he may no longer be able to maintain the focus tension required for distant viewing that a normal subject would use when looking at an object three inches away.

Farsightedness is by far a worse impairment than nearsightedness. When patients ask me, as they often do, "please make me farsighted rather than nearsighted," they do not know what they are asking. It's a little like saying, "I have a bad limp; can you cut my leg off so I won't limp anymore?" If only one thing comes from writing this book, I hope it is that people will not think farsightedness is preferable to nearsightedness.

Is Radial Keratotomy Safe?

The Risk of Unpredictable Results with RK: the PERK Study*

When RK was in its infancy in this country, the National Institute of Health decided to sponsor a major research project to be carried out by several prominent investigators at different locations across America. The study was designed in such a way so that the surgery would attempt to correct the patient's visual handicap to produce normal vision with the most consistent results, results which would be studied over a period of three years. While you may read the study for yourself, let me say that the results of this study are somewhat discouraging; discouraging on a number of counts. The study concludes that there is "considerable inherent surgical and biological variability in radial keratotomy." That is to say that the state of the art examined by this study could not identify with any predictable accuracy the nature of the correction which would be achieved by the surgery. So, inevitably some eyes would be overcorrected and some undercorrected.

> PATIENTS OLDER THAN FORTY RUN A GREATER RISK OF OVER-REACTING TO THE SURGERY TO THE POINT OF REMAINING FARSIGHTED.

While the information gleaned from this study has been very valuable, and still constitutes one of the major bodies of research into RK in this country, it must be observed that two very significant variables were omitted from the scientific evaluation: the age and sex of the patients. As part of the methodology of

53

the study, each operation undertaken by members of the PERK team seems to have been very rigidly performed according to the design of the study. So for example, each surgery was begun by imprinting a circle on the cornea directly over the pupil. All incisions were to reach from the edge of the cornea to touch this circle without entering it. Thus, the smaller the circle, the longer the incisions, and the greater the amount of correction. As a result they took a group of patients who had been selected because they had a certain degree of myopia and did the same operation on each of them. No modification was made which would have lengthened the incisions for younger subjects or shortened them in older patients. In addition, no adjustment was made to account for sex differences.

> A SIGNIFICANT NUMBER OF PATIENTS BECOME TEMPORARILY FARSIGHTED AFTER SURGERY, MAKING IT DIFFICULT TO DO A GREAT DEAL OF CLOSEUP WORK FOR SOME TIME.

Many RK surgeons regularly take these factors into consideration and make adjustments in their procedure as a consequence. The rigidity of the design of this study did not allow for them even after the need for such adjustments became obvious. [For a similar study see "Michael R. Deitz, M.D., and others, "Consecutive Series (1982-1985) of Radial Keratotomies Performed with the Diamond Blade," *American Journal of Ophthalmology,* 103 (March 1987), 417-22.]

Is Radial Keratotomy Safe?

Figure 7: Each Surgery Is Begun By Imprinting a Circle on the Cornea Directly Over the Pupil.

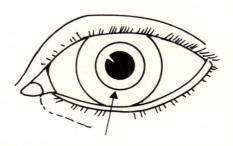

The PERK study is still highly regarded by the medical profession so it is important that you have access to it. The professionals who conducted the PERK study are all very distinguished and important surgeons for whom the American Medical Association and the American Academy of Ophthalmology and I have great respect. Their contribution to the understanding of RK is substantial, and I do not mean to detract from their obvious achievements, but at the same time I want you to know that on this issue of predictability—which is one of the most serious limitations of RK often cited in the popular press—I have had a very different experience in my own practice. [There is a significant controversy revolving around the bad press stimulated by the PERK study as typified by "Goodbye Glasses?" *Consumer Reports,* 53:1 (January 1988), 52-4; see especially "Clinical Trial Stirs Legal Battles" *Science,* 227 (March 15, 1985), 1316.]

My Methods for Increasing the Predictability of RK
I regard RK as a two-stage operation. In other words, my patients know before having the surgery

that there is a possibility that two operations will need to be done for each eye. I aim for a ninety percent correction of each patient's nearsightedness. Frequently, a patient will return for his followup examination and I will discover that I have given him a one hundred percent correction. From these patients, needless to say, I have had few complaints.

Most of the group of patients who remain are ninety percent corrected. Their vision will be in the 20/30 to 20/25 range, enabling them to function well at all tasks involving distant vision without glasses. The complaint I hear most often is that driving at night in an unfamiliar area is worrisome. A person who is slightly nearsighted after RK surgery will see his best upon awakening, whatever the hour may be. For most individuals who rise in the morning and sleep in the nighttime, this means that clarity of vision will decrease somewhat during the latter part of their day. This puts the time of decreased visual acuity at night. When a patient discovers this circumstance, I advise them to wait at least six months before a second surgery. I find this a useful precaution because very often some of these patients will find their eyes correcting themselves after this period of time. I will recommend the second surgery for this group of patients, if I think it is safe and if meaningful gains are reasonably to be anticipated. It should be noted that I have not seen a shift toward farsightedness with the passage of time to any significant degree in my patients after four years of performing this operation. The PERK study has predicted such a shift, so I continue to watch for it.

About twenty percent of my patients require a second operation because of undercorrection. I believe

Is Radial Keratotomy Safe?

that I could decrease this percentage easily by making longer incisions, but I would risk overcorrecting an approximate ten percent of my patients. For me, that risk is too high! Hence, I plod along with a two-stage surgical procedure.

> IT MAY TAKE SEVERAL DAYS FOR NORMAL VISUAL ACUITY TO BE ACHIEVED. IN SOME EXTREME CASES UP TO SIX MONTHS HAVE BEEN NECESSARY FOR STABILIZATION OF VISION.

To date, I have experienced only two cases of overcorrection among the more than two thousand operations performed. Even though their degree of overcorrection is not severe, and they represent less than 0.1 percent of my RK case history records, I have been moved to take great pains to minimize the risk of overcorrection as a result of their situations.

The Risk of Cataract Formation as a Result of RK

Another possible complication of RK is cataract formation. As we saw in Chapter Three, a cataract is a clouding of the crystalline lens which lies directly behind the cornea, the aqueous humour and the iris. To date this is treatable only by surgical removal of the crystalline lens. From my reading of the published literature, I know of six instances in which RK surgery has caused cataracts. It used to be thought that placing the eye under great pressure during surgery would cause the correction sought by the surgeon performing RK to be greater. In three cases, when the perforation of the cornea occurred, the pressure collapsed the lens toward the surgeon's scalpel. The slightest nick of this exquisitely sensitive tissue results in a cataract. The other three cases were caused by prolonged exposure of the eye to steroids contained in cortisone eye drops prescribed after RK surgery in an attempt to achieve greater correction. In each of these six cases the surgeon was trying to achieve greater corrections than the usual RK parameters permit: these techniques have now been largely abandoned, and I have never used them.

The Risk of Losing the Protection of Glasses
Some of my patients have voiced the fear that their eyes would get hurt in the process of daily activity if they did not wear glasses. And I can understand this fear because I can think of several instances when I had an accident in which my glasses hit a tree limb and when I was thankful that I had them on.

However, during my years of experience with RK, no patient has sustained a significant injury to an eye following surgery. This defies common sense, I know, and I have no authoritative explanation. On the other hand, I have treated many eye injuries for patients wearing glasses or contact lenses at the time of the trauma.

I wish to emphasize very strongly here that the wearing of safety glasses is an absolute requirement of certain occupations, as well as some hobbies. Having RK surgery does not relieve a patient from the obligation to care for his eyes in the presence of danger, including, but not limited to, driving nails, using a grindstone, power saw or mower—any activity which might cause a high-speed projectile to travel toward the eye. One mistake could cause a blinding injury.

Is Radial Keratotomy Safe?

The Risk of Corneal Scarring Caused by RK

The latest popular objection I have heard concerns the risk of permanent scarring of the cornea. The truth about these scars is that:

- The corneal scars which result from RK are one tenth of a millimeter wide, and about three millimeters long; there are usually eight per eye.
- The scars gradually fade,until after three years I can no longer see them under a microscope.

Regardless of what some well meaning individuals may tell you:

- The scars do not merge over time.
- The scars do not turn cloudy.
- The scars are not recognizable and do not cause any observable disfiguration.

The Risk of Losing Visual Acuity

Some of my patients have voiced the fear of losing visual acuity after RK. By this they mean that even with glasses they fear they would be unable to see as well as they could before the surgery. This same concern is voiced by the PERK Study. I have never seen this in any of my patients, but from my reading of the medical literature, I believe it may be caused by some form of irregular astigmatism induced by the surgery. Obviously, such a problem might have a variety of origins, one being the failure to properly center the surgery with the line of vision. I cannot speak with authority about this complication, but its incidence is small and should continue to decrease as the profession gains experience with RK.

The Risk of Retinal Detachment

One of my patients had a retinal detachment following RK. She had a small hole in the retina when I examined her initially, and as about eight percent of the population have such a problem and never go on to have retinal detachments, I completed the surgery. After the detachment, it was determined that RK was not a contributing factor to it, and it was repaired successfully. This patient still has 20/20 vision in that eye, without glasses.

What Is the Long Term Effect of RK?

Perhaps the greatest concern and most legitimate one a patient may ask is what will happen forty years from now, if he/she has this operation? Since the American experience with this operation is less than fifteen years, it is obvious that no one can now provide a suitable answer to this question. There are tests we can run, from which we can develop a probable projection, but let's face it, no one can be certain.

Remember that in Chapter Two and again in Chapter Three we described the cornea's endothelial layer? This layer is only one cell thick and lies on the underside of the cornea where it functions to pump water out of the cornea and thereby maintains the vital partial dehydration of the cornea which is necessary if it is to retain its transparency. When one cell of this layer is damaged it cannot replace itself, so when it dies its neighbors widen and flatten to occupy its space, so that none of the interior cornea remains unlined. The result is that as we get older these cells decrease in number, and the remaining cells become deformed, exhibiting a great variety in size and shape. We can measure this variability. [See Setsuko, M. D., and others, "Risk Factors in Radial Keratotomy," *Journal of Cataract and Refractive Surgery,* 13 (1987), 263-7.] We can even photograph and document changes in this layer. After fifteen years of case histories involving RK, there is no conclusive evidence that any damage is done to these cells by RK. The same cannot be said of contact lenses. Wearing hard contact lenses causes severe and permanent damage to this endothelial layer. Even soft contact lenses damage this layer, although less so than hard contacts. [See Scott M. Mac Rae, M.D., and others "The Effects of Hard and Soft Contact Lenses on the Corneal Endothelium," *American Journal of Ophthalmology,* 102:1 (July 1986), 50-57.]

If I thought that RK could cause as much damage to the endothelium as soft contact lenses do, I would cease performing the operation, and society at large would probably demand its termination. Ironically, no such hue and cry arises about the damage contacts cause to this vital tissue. I have often wondered why this is so. What causes the double standard here so demonstrably present in the public and professional acceptance of contacts and the public resistance to RK, which has not even shown a hint of damaging this all important tissue?

As I observed in Chapter Two, my chief concern over the damage to this tissue is the long term effect of such damage added to that of cataract surgery. I have to wonder if when my patients grow older and require

I Can See!

cataract surgery, as many of the elderly will do, what effect the RK operation will have on their cataract operation. Will they be better off than their peers who wore contacts from their youth? In my opinion, they certainly will be, but only time will tell. So far only a few RK patients have had cataract surgery and have done very well, but there is not enough evidence here to permit me to draw any valid conclusion in this regard.

These are the risks which I have heard voiced most often by my patients. I must say that in the final analysis none of these risks prevented me from having the surgery, on my own eyes. In my particular case, at age forty-five, in my profession as eye surgeon I had one other consideration. I feared giving up my near vision, as it is vital to my work. Most of the time during surgery my face is less than one foot from my patient's eye. I chose to have one eye fully corrected for distant vision, while the other was undercorrected to allow me to see well at close range. This peculiar adaptation of RK works wonderfully for me, but it would not be tolerated by most patients.

*[Permission to reprint the article by George O. Waring, M.D. and others, "Three-year Results of the Prospective Evaluation of Radial Keratotomy (PERK) Study," *Ophthalmology*, Volume 94, Number 10 (October 1987), 1339-1354 as an appendix in this book was denied after *I Can See!* had gone to Press.

Although J. B. Lippincott/Harper and Row, *Ophthalmology's* publisher, sold a license to Osler House, the Editor-in-Chief of *Ophthalmology* refused permission: "It is not our policy to waive copyright in order to allow articles that have been published in *Ophthalmology* to appear in the lay press. As you know, material in this journal is quite technical. It is written by and for

Is Radial Keratotomy Safe?

ophthalmologists or basic science researchers whose work pertains to ophthalmology. Therefore, we do not grant you permission to reprint Dr. Waring's October article on the PERK Study." This letter was sent by Paul R. Lichter, M.D.;address: W. K. Kellogg Eye Center, 1000 Wall Street, Ann Arbor, MI 48105-1910.]

5

Will Radial Keratotomy Help You?

I receive many calls from people who hope that RK might improve their ability to read. For the most part, these individuals have never really had difficulty with their vision until about the age of forty-five, then suddenly they discover that they are unable to read without glasses. My answer usually is that RK is not the solution to this particular problem, but there may be other ways to resolve it, ways beyond the scope of this particular book.

RK is not a cure for the aging process. This is a crucial realization, and I cannot stress it too strongly. RK surgery will not help you recover the visual capacity of your youth!!! On the contrary, I can promise that in all likelihood you will need reading glasses after the age of forty-five. If you have RK you will become a normal person who is subject to all the frailties of normal people.

It is the rare myope who does not love to read or who does not derive a great deal of pleasure from reading. Most who come to me for consultation can read

I Can See!

very well without glasses, and these people find it very difficult to accept that after RK they will have to wear glasses to read. If your greatest pleasure comes from reading and you are over forty, then you should think long and hard about having RK surgery for it will most certainly remove the good near vision necessary for an unaided reading ability.

What Optical Handicaps Are Correctable by RK?

If you are nearsighted you can see things close up better than you can see things far off. If you are able to drive your car without glasses, you probably do not need this operation. If you can read at a comfortable distance without glasses, but cannot see well in the distance, you may be a perfect candidate for RK.

READING GLASSES MAY BE REQUIRED PERMANENTLY AFTER THE SURGERY, ESPECIALLY IN PATIENTS OVER FORTY YEARS OF AGE

The Newspaper Test

You can get some idea of the extent of your myopia by doing a simple test we call the "Newspaper Test."

Step One: If you wear glasses or contact lenses, remove them.

Step Two: Hold a newspaper one inch from your nose.

Step Three: Gradually move the newspaper away from your nose until your eyes can render the ordinary sized newsprint readable. The distance established in this manner is called your near point of vision.

Step Four: Now move the newspaper away from your face farther until the print begins to blur. You may discover that you have to place the newspaper on a dresser or bookcase in order to achieve this distance. The distance established in this manner is called your far point of vision.

Step Five: Now measure the distance from your eye brow to the print.

RESULTS: If, when you measure the far point of vision, you obtain a measurement between eight inches and forty inches, your odds of achieving good vision after RK surgery without glasses are very high. If your far point of vision is less than eight inches away, you will not be able to get 20/20 vision through RK surgery, with a few exceptions. One of these exceptions includes people who are well over forty years of age.

Significant astigmatism will make the newspaper test impossible to perform.

Age and Sex Differences

It is possible to produce more correction with RK in older patients probably because the body has a natural tendency, which decreases with age, to overcome the surgery. The operation is less extensive in older individuals. At the other end of the spectrum are teenagers. It is very difficult to achieve a full correction on eighteen-year-olds, especially eighteen-year-old

women. For some reason, it usually takes more surgery to correct the visual handicap of females than of
men of the same age.

A Technical Definition: The Diopter
    A diopter is the unit of measurement most often
applied to myopic vision, and we obtain this measurement by knowing the far point of vision, in metric
terms.
    Let us assume that in a given case the far point lies
at fifty centimeters (1/2 meter) from the eye. Once we
have this fraction, we invert it and thus the reading of
two diopters describes the degree of this patient's visual disability. We use a plus or minus sign to indicate
whether the condition measured is nearsightedness or
farsightedness. A minus sign (-) indicates myopia and
a plus sign (+) indicates hyperopia. In this case the
myopic eye is described as "-2." You can perform this
same calculation for other sets of numbers. Suppose
the far point was at two meters. This would be written
as the fraction 2/1 meters. Again, by inverting, just as
in our other fraction, we have 1/2 diopter. We use the
decimal equivalent or 0.5 diopter to designate this
person's eyeglass prescription. The number is mean-
ingless unless we say "-0.5 diopters." Similarly, if
there were no refractive error in your eye, then we
might say you could wear glasses with a power of zero
diopters, that is to say window glass.
    Using this terminology then, we can say that RK
surgery is most successful for patients whose visual
handicaps may be described as existing on a range of
visual impairment between -0.5 diopters and -5.0 diopters. Put another way, we might say that if the far
point of your vision is found to be between two meters

Will Radial Keratotomy Help You?

and twenty centimeters (one-fifth of a meter) then RK will probably help you. Such a range takes care of most nearsighted patients, as those with higher degrees of myopia are unusual. The limits of RK are such that if your far point is closer than one-fifth meter away, you will likely require glasses even after having the surgery. The limitations of correction from RK are about five diopters in a young person, while up to eight diopters of correction are possible after age fifty.

A Technical Description: Normal Versus Abnormal Vision

The concept of vision as rays of light entering the eye is not easy to grasp. Think of a tiny point of illumination which projects light in all directions. This light is composed of billions of light rays and that the distance between light rays grows wider as they leave the source of illumination. Now move the light source farther away from the eye. The divergence of incoming light rays grows smaller. If we could move the light source out to infinity, these rays would be parallel to each other. In the special world of visual optics, "infinity" occurs at about twenty feet away, where, for all practical purposes the light rays are considered to have become parallel. This is an important distance, one that has led us to evaluate distance vision in terms of what we all know as the famous index of normal vision, 20/20 vision. 20/20 vision simply means that the normal individual can see a standardized amount of detail clearly at twenty feet. A patient who has 20/40 vision can see at twenty feet what the normal person sees at forty feet.

69

I Can See!

Figure 8: The Point of Focus in a Normal or Emmetropic Eye Falls Directly upon the Retina.

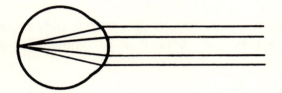

The Function of the Myopic Eye

Now suppose that the light source is twenty feet away. The light rays are gradually getting farther apart as they move out towards the horizon. To do more than merely register that light is present, as some photorective organs in protozoa do, the human eye has to bend the light rays back towards each other so they come to a point upon the retina. Bending light this way is called refraction. When this occurs, the light is said to be in clear focus. We have seen that this bending action is accomplished by the cooperation of the cornea and the crystalline lens. The greater the curvature of the cornea, the more bending of the light will occur. Suppose now that the cornea is curved too sharply. The rays will be bent in too much and the point of focus will fall short of the retina. The image cast by this convergence of light will be blurred as the light rays diverge once more by the time they reach the retina.

Will Radial Keratotomy Help You?

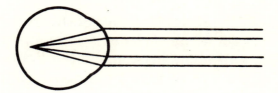

Figure 9: The Point of Focus in a Myopic or Nearsighted Eye Falls in Front of the Retina.

When the eye is focusing light so that it falls short of the retina, the resultant blurred vision is called myopia or nearsightedness. We can see that by moving the light source closer to the eye, we soon reach a point where the distance between the light rays and the power of the cornea to bend them is exactly sufficient to place the image in focus upon the retina. This distance from the cornea to the light source is called the far point and represents for that individual in question the maximum distance possible for sharp vision.

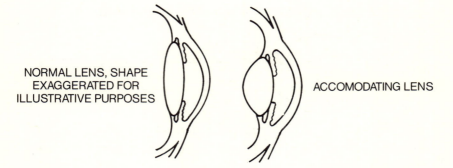

NORMAL LENS, SHAPE EXAGGERATED FOR ILLUSTRATIVE PURPOSES

ACCOMODATING LENS

Figure 10: In Accommodation the Lens of the Normal Eye (Drawn Here in an Exaggerated Thinness for Illustrative Purposes at Left) Changes Shape in an Attempt to Bring the Object of Regard into Focus.

I Can See!

The lens in its oval resting state contributes about forty percent of the refractive power of the cornea. Accommodation, or rounding of the lens through its own focusing effort, will allow us to move the light source even closer to the eye and still maintain this sharp retinal image.

Many nearsighted persons have a far point which is exactly proper for reading—about eighteen inches or so from the eye. It is possible for them to read without exerting any focusing effort whatever. No matter how old they become, if all else remains well, they will always be able to read without glasses, but distance vision will always be poor if no corrective device is worn or no corrective surgery is performed.

What if the cornea has the proper curve, but the eye grows too much, creating a greater distance from the front to back? This also results in myopia since the light rays focus sharply in front of the retina. I have seen some patients who have eyes that are too long and corneas that are too curved. These individuals may have severe myopia which requires glasses resembling telescopes for adequate correction.

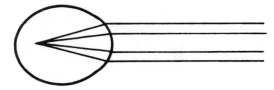

Figure 11: Myopia May Also be Caused by an Eye with a Normal Cornea but with an Unusually Lengthened General Eye Structure.

Will Radial Keratotomy Help You?

The Functioning of the Farsighted Eye, or the Eye Afflicted with Hyperopia

Conversely, if the cornea is not curved enough, the light rays will be poorly bent so that they have not converged to a point by the time the light reaches the retina. This condition is called hyperopia or farsightedness. Hyperopia may also be caused by an eye which is small, or short, and it may be quite severe.

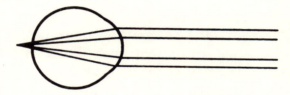

Figure 12: In a Farsighted Eye or Hyperopic Eye the Point of Focus Falls Behind the Retina.

Look at the illustrations and try to understand this point: a person may be farsighted and yet function very well during childhood, because he can use the focusing power of the crystalline lens to add more bending to the light rays entering his eye. No such option is available for the myope. He MUST wear correction to see well in the distance. However, as the hyperope becomes older, he will reach the point where he can no longer focus enough with the crystalline lens to do this adequately, thus he will also need glasses. Before this age the farsighted person will already have noticed that he cannot read well . . . he is using all his

73

focusing power to see in the distance and has none left for near viewing.

I have heard many people speak of farsightedness with great respect. Some will say, for example: "I'd rather be farsighted than nearsighted." Such people do not realize the disadvantage that hyperopia causes in later life. Severe headaches can result, first when reading, then later almost constantly as the lens becomes less able to provide the refraction they need.

The Emmetrope or Normally Sighted Person

The person who is neither nearsighted nor farsighted is called an emmetrope. These are the fortunate ones, and they constitute at least sixty-five percent of the population. Their visual problems begin at about age forty-five, when their lens also begins to lose its ability to accommodate and they begin holding materials farther away in order to read them. This condition is called presbyopia. It is corrected by wearing farsighted glasses while reading. If one has either nearsightedness or farsightedness, he eventually resorts to wearing bifocal eyeglasses as he grows older; the upper portion of such glasses are used to see at a distance while the lower segment is used for reading or other close work.

Astigmatism

Let us consider the special case of *astigmatism.* Suppose that the eye were a basketball, and that the basketball was made in such a way so that half of it were transparent, and the remaining half were opaque. Let the opaque half represent the portion of the globe of the eye taken up by the delicate sensors of the retina, while the transparent half represents the

Will Radial Keratotomy Help You?

part of the eye facing the external world, upon which surface you would find the cornea. Now if pressure were applied to the top and bottom of the basketball in this model of the eye, a distortion of the cornea would take place. The globe would be flatter on the top and bottom of its cap-like shape while the curve of its surface nearest the nose and temple would be more extreme. This is approximately the problem presented by astigmatism. Astigmatism is the cause of many headaches as the internal muscles of the eye try to alter the image in order to compensate for distortion. Astigmatism is difficult to correct with glasses. Hard contact lenses are more helpful, as they give the front of the eye a more uniformly curved surface.

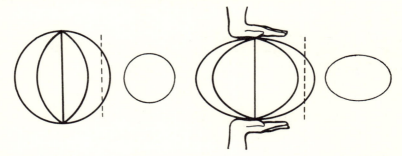

Figure 13: In Order to Understand Astigmatism It May Help to Compare the Eye to a Basketball. In a Normal Eye, the Cornea is Circular, like the Forward Section of this Basketball. In the Astigmatic Eye, the Cornea is Oval in the Same Way that the Forward Section of This Basketball Would be if Pressure Were Applied to Top and Bottom.

RK helps astigmatism by selectively changing the shape of the cornea in only one direction. Ideally some myopia should also be present if the surgery is to work most successfully, but in general this is the corner-stone of astigmatic surgery. RK will help myopia and no other condition, except in certain cases of astigmatism. The effect of RK is to cause the curvature of the central cornea to flatten, thus the corneal surface is capable of less refraction. It is effective in either the type of nearsightedness caused by too great a curve of the cornea or that type caused by an eye that is too long. However, I believe that RK works slightly better in cases of increased corneal curvature.

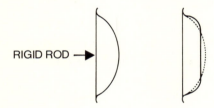

RIGID ROD →

Figure 14: The Cornea of the Normal Eye, Seen in a Cross-Section Is Like This Bow. After RK the Shape of the Cornea Is Flatter Like This Second Bow.

Let me propose another model for you. Imagine that hanging on your wall is an archer's bow. Someone has replaced the string with an unbendable steel rod. The only portion of the bow that will bend is the wooden part. Place your hand in the middle of the bow and push it towards the steel rod. What happens? The curve of the bow becomes flatter in the middle, but steeper at the top and bottom. Conversely, if you place your hands farther apart near the ends of the bow and pull the ends away from each other, the middle will become flatter. This is exactly how RK surgery works . . . it makes the center of the cornea flatter by making the rest of it more curved.

Will Radial Keratotomy Help You?

Staphyloma

Staphyloma is a special and very rare type of near-sightedness and is caused by a progressive bulging of the back of the eye. If RK is done for such a patient, it may help greatly for a time, but later correction might prove to be insufficient as the retina gets farther away from the cornea.

Current thinking is that RK should not be performed on an eye which has a vision threatening disorder, such as uncontrollable glaucoma, or in cases of severe diabetes, corneal dystrophies and degenerations, or recurrent severe corneal infections. A repaired retinal detachment may create myopia which may be helped by RK, but I am not exactly eager to perform RK on such individuals. I have never performed RK on a patient with only one seeing eye.

Nystagmus

Nystagmus is the term used to designate rapid, involuntary eye movements. This condition is usually accompanied by some degree of poor vision, even when the best possible eyeglasses are worn. RK will not fully correct the vision of these patients.

Progressive Degenerative Myopia

Progressive degenerative myopia cannot be arrested by RK. If the process which has caused your myopia has not reached conclusion then you will continue to become more myopic until it does reach conclusion. RK will only let you start the process over at a less myopic point. For this reason I do not perform RK on individuals younger than eighteen years of age, and then I consider it only if their myopia has gotten

77

I Can See!

no worse during the year immediately preceding.

In general, if vision cannot be corrected to 20/20 by eyeglasses or contact lenses, it will not usually be possible to get this correction by RK either. Myopia in the presence of even very mild cataracts should not be corrected by RK, as cataract lens implant surgery will eventually be necessary anyway, and the power of the implant can be selected to correct the myopia without putting the patient through a needless separate operation (RK).

6

The Surgery and How to Prepare for It

Let's assume, for whatever reasons, you have decided to have RK performed on your eyes.

How to Find an RK Surgeon

Your first challenge is to find the surgeon to whom you are going to entrust the correction of your vision. After you have read the next chapter on the controversy surrounding RK, you will have a better understanding of what kind of biases you will encounter as you search for recommendations.

What I would like to do is to recommend a pattern of criteria and sources which in my opinion will provide you with a reasonable chance of developing enough information to permit you to make an informed decision.

In the most general terms, there are several sources from which you may develop a list of surgeons in your region who perform RK.

1) Of course, there are the trusty yellow pages wherein physicians may indicate that RK is one of their specialties.

2) You may call or write to the American Society of Cataract and Refractive Surgery, 3702 Pender Drive, Suite 250, Fairfax, Va. 22030, Phone: (703) 591-2202.

3) A variety of reference services may exist in your city, such as the local medical society or the hospital referral service.

4) If you have an ophthalmologist from whom you have been receiving treatment or regular checkups, you certainly should seek his or her advice in such a matter.

Many physicians who perform RK surgery have found to their chagrin that not only do their colleagues who do not perform the surgery advise their patients against it, but they will actually deny the existence of any local RK surgeons. Persistence in calling all local eye surgeons will usually pay off in such a situation, and you will discover the specialists who deliver this vision enhancing surgery to their patients.

Why Are There So Few RK Surgeons?
I have seen many doctors who decide that perhaps RK is a good thing, and who consequently attend one or more of the courses given regularly by one of the various RK specialists. These courses of study may include a series of lectures and films and perhaps even an opportunity to watch the surgery performed. When these individuals return home with the hope of including this surgery in their repertoire of surgical procedures which will aid their patients, one of their first tasks will be to investigate the availability of hospital facilities in which the surgery might be practiced. Many, if not most, of them will discover that their local hospitals have already made the decision not to equip

80

The Surgery and How to Prepare for It

their operating rooms with the expensive equipment required before even the first incision can be made. This in and of itself stops ninety percent of such surgeons in their tracks, as their only alternative is to set up their own facility at their own expense. In the fast moving world of surgical equipment, technology waits for no surgeon. Not only will they have to have the financial ability to equip their own operating room, but they must be willing to commit the financial resources to updating their equipment as the technology becomes more refined and advanced. Such a commitment to a procedure whose practitioners are so caught up in controversy is a challenging decision which takes a lot of courage and self-confidence. By definition then RK surgeons who have made the decision are a breed apart and may represent only ten percent of all those who have considered the possibility.

Once the decision to embrace RK as part of a surgeon's practice has been made there is always the temptation to try to economize on what tools will be acquired. And some may discover that they have established their surgery with equipment which will not permit them to do their best work. In RK surgery the highest quality work requires the most sophisticated technology available.

But let's say that the RK surgeon has equipped his surgery with the best equipment money will buy. Now comes the time to do the first operation. Take it from one who knows, the entire future of a potential RK surgeon depends on the outcome of the first twenty cases. Although skill and equipment are crucial factors in the success of these cases, luck may play a higher role than any of us would like to admit.

I Can See!

Only about half of those who have reached this stage will actually do their first surgery because they suddenly come face to face with intelligent questions from patients who want the operation or who have had the operation. An RK surgeon must be part educator, part psychologist because he must work with the very real fears and anxieties of patients who may be perceptually handicapped but who are very often intellectually gifted. I discover that I spend about fifteen percent of my day counseling patients, and I realize that this is a significant part of my interaction with these individuals who have come to me with the hope that medical science has at long last found a way to resolve their visual handicaps. To be candid, this is one reason I have taken the time to write this book: *I want my patients to know RK inside and out, and I can answer many general knowledge questions here. In this way I can focus in more detail on patient-specific issues as I encounter them.*

One Measure of a Good RK Surgeon

As with any surgery, one of the criteria which distinguishes a successful practitioner is the frequency with which he performs the procedure. When I went looking for a surgeon to do my RK surgery, I looked for someone who did a lot of RK surgery. Such surgeons have paid the price. They have had enough faith in themselves to devote most of their time to the special problems of RK patients, and they have achieved a quantifiable measure of success or they would not have such self-confidence. There can be no better recommendation than success, because if an RK surgeon cannot produce, he will not maintain his practice.

The Surgery and How to Prepare for It

The Self-Advertising Phobia

As we have seen, for the RK surgeon the traditional method of receiving patients by means of referrals from other ophthalmologists and physicians is blocked by much of the controversy with which RK has been saddled. Consequently, many RK surgeons have been forced to advertise their presence in the medical community by resorting to the media. In a profession as conservative as medicine, the decision to advertise is a difficult one because we physicians often do not like to admit that we are part of a competitive trade, one where access to patients may be blocked by professional disputes and marketing jealousies. For RK surgeons advertising is often a requirement, not a luxury. In the pursuit of an RK surgeon, you should not be put off by public announcements of his services.

References

The physician you select may be open to a request for patient references. There can be no better confirmation of a physician's skill than the testimony of satisfied patients. As the number of patients who have had this surgery grows—and that is one of the certainties of radial keratotomy—it will not be difficult to locate individuals who either have had the surgery or know of friends or relatives who have had it. Very often physicians may refuse to provide you with the names of patients who have had the surgery, as the relationship between a patient and his or her physician is protected by both medical ethics and legal statutes. But persistence will usually reward you with direct testimony of more than one patient who can give you the "scoop" on the operation.

I Can See!

The Issue of Compatibility

It is crucial that you have confidence in the surgeon who is to perform your surgery. If you have not, if you have what they call in detective novels a "gut" feeling that says, "Don't go with this guy," don't! You must be comfortable with every significant aspect of your surgery. If you are not able to relax when the time comes for your surgery because of lack of trust, you are inviting trouble.

The Issue of Fees

Ask your surgeon about the fees for this procedure. This is elective surgery, and there is no reason you should not be as completely informed about the fiscal aspects of the surgery as you are about the physical aspects. Here are some of the questions you might ask:

- Will both eyes be operated on at the same time?
- Is there a separate fee for each surgery or one fee for both?
- Is there an additional fee for use of the operating room?
- Is the procedure covered by insurance?
- If the procedure should need to be repeated, does the second operation on each eye cost extra?
- What is the cost of the follow-up visits?

A Radial Keratotomy Guide

Let us assume that you have elected to have the surgery, and that you have decided on which surgeon you would like to perform the surgery. At this stage each surgeon will have his own established procedures. Each of us finds one set of practices which is most successful, so if the surgeon you have selected has a variant of the following step guide you should not be surprised. Since I designed this book from my own experience, it makes sense that I should record here my surgical step guide. However, for my readers across the nation who find a fellow ophthalmologist more convenient I would hasten to assure them that what follows is not the only procedure which will produce good results.

My Preferences

As you may have surmised, my preference is to operate on both eyes at one sitting, unless the patient has a strong misgiving about it. Most RK surgeons prefer to operate on one eye at a time. The rationale most often given for this serial routine is that they want to have the opportunity to judge the effect of the surgery on the first eye so that any necessary adjustment could be made for the second eye. The fallacy I discovered in this reasoning lies in the fact that most patients will want the second eye operated on far in advance of the time frame in which this knowledge will become available.

However, each surgeon will have established his or her own routine, and once they have met success within that routine they will be very reluctant to break their own rules. I don't argue with them at all.

I have observed that the most common complaint following surgery on the first eye was not discomfort, glare, or tear excess, but the discomfort caused by the visual unequalization between the two eyes. It is common practice for plastic surgeons to undertake cosmetic eyelid surgery on both sides simultaneously, and that operation carries a risk of blindness at least as great as that for RK. Few ask the plastic surgeons to fix only one eyelid at a time because it would be very difficult to make the eyelids match each other unless both are done at the same time.

Furthermore it is inescapable that there is a certain amount of discomfort following RK surgery, and this discomfort may last from two to four days. Why ask RK patients to endure this uncomfortable period twice? My experience has been that those patients on whom I have operated one eye at a time have invariably said they wished they had gotten the whole process finished in one sitting. And no patient upon whom I have operated on both eyes at once has ever expressed regret of any kind that this was the procedure. My preference to do both eyes at once works for me, but it is not the preference of all RK surgeons. Please do not expect your surgeon of choice to violate his own preference should he or she wish to operate on each eye separately. In my own case, I had to fly to California on two separate occasions to complete my RK surgeries. I'd do it exactly that way again, without hesitation.

Personal Hygiene in the Days Just Before the Surgery
EYEDROPS: When a specific date and hour of the day is established for your operation, I will ask you to use a special eyedrop in your eyes during the two days before you present yourself at the surgery.

CONTACT LENSES: If you regularly wear contact lenses, I will ask you to leave them out for the same period of time. In this way, your body will have time to repair any minor damage to the delicate corneal surfaces caused by wearing contact lenses. The oxygen deficiency in these tissues (or minor abrasions or traumas such lens wear may cause) will usually be corrected by this period of restoration.

COSMETICS: I ask all my female patients to cease wearing eye makeup the night before surgery and to clean thoroughly all cosmetics from the eyelids and eyelashes. You cannot imagine how wonderfully bacteria grow in such cosmetic preparations. (See Louis Wilson, and others, "The Survival and Growth of Microorganisms in Mascara During Use," *American Journal of Ophthalmology,* 79:4 (April 1975), 596-600.) Should any of this material find its way into your incisions it will remain there forever and become a fertile ground in which bacteria will grow without restraint. This we do not need!

Getting Ready for the Day of Your Surgery

FOOD AND DRINK: Many surgeons who perform RK request that you do not drink or eat after midnight before the day of your surgery. There are many reasons for this, but in many institutions it is required in the by-laws of the medical staff. My patients are allowed, even encouraged, to eat breakfast on the morning of surgery. The dual misery of hunger and postoperative discomfort is unnecessary.

SEDATION: I have had patients present themselves for surgery in nearly every state of sedation imaginable. Some arrive intoxicated by alcohol, others come—as we used to say in the sixties—"stoned" or heavily drugged.

I Can See!

Please come to the surgery without preparing your-self with such chemical assists. It is very dangerous to have drugs in your system which your surgeon may not have prescribed or be aware of. Your surgeon will be administering some very potent drugs to you during and after the surgery, and there is considerable danger of these drugs reacting with those you may have taken without his knowledge.

Remember, this is elective surgery: it is not supposed to be life threatening!

On the Day of the Surgery
In other times, surgery such as this would have required several days of hospitalization. But today it is a one day event, and you will sleep in a bed of your own choosing. As you will not drive yourself home from this operation, it is important that you make some arrangements with family or friends to bring you to the surgery and return you home that night. You will be taking some pretty strong medication which will temporarily impair your judgment and your reaction time.

Furthermore, you should not plan to make any important business decisions during the next two days, as it will take this long for the medication to wear off.

The "Which Eye Are We Operating on Today?"
Questions
Throughout the day, you will hear seemingly a hundred times "Which eye are we operating on today?" You would think we would know all this, but you cannot imagine how easy it is to operate on the wrong eye. Please do not take offense at such questions. A

moment of carelessness, a heavily sedated patient, it only takes five minutes to do irreparable harm. So let them ask, hope they ask you—and for God's sake give them the same answer each time. All levity aside, if they don't ask this question, volunteer the information with some regularity.

Special Clothing

The clothing you wear in from the street may not be suitable for operating room conditions. Some surgeons will require that you remove your clothing and put on a special gown. Other surgeons—among which I count myself—will simply isolate the field of the operation with sterile surgical drapery, and proceed.

Anesthetizing the Eye

The usual means of anesthetizing the eye is to use drops in repeated doses, which provide a temporary but profound effect so that no pain is felt. Additional medication may be applied by cotton applicators used around the edge of the cornea, so that you will not feel the device used to immobilize the eye.

Immobilizing the Head

During the entire operation the surgeon's hands will rest against your forehead or face in such a way that if you make any sudden head movements, his hands will move with you. A sudden sneeze could be catastrophic otherwise.

Obviously, when in the course of the operation his hand is on your chin or mouth, it would be advisable not to speak or smile. Usually this is not a problem given the state of sedation you will enter.

I Can See!

Creating the Sterile Field Around the Area of the Operation

Your face will be washed with a germicidal soap which will not injure your eye. A sterile drape will be placed over your head so that nothing is exposed except your eye. A great deal of effort and caution to produce a sterile state on instruments is used to ensure that the possibility of infection is minimized. Although I have read in the literature that some surgeons sterilize their knives by soaking them in a metal tray containing acetone, I have never done so. Lucky for me that I didn't, as sometime later I read reports that a peculiar type of corneal infection related to the tuberculosis bacteria which sometimes occasioned the RK surgery was somehow related to this acetone sterilization procedure. ["Mycobacterium Cheloni Keratitis After Radial Keratotomy." *American Journal of Ophthalmology.* 102 (July 1986), 72-79.] In some ways I'm a little old fashioned, so I have always used a full sized hospital-grade autoclave to sterilize all instruments and surgical linens.

Immobilizing the Eye Itself

A device called the speculum is placed between the eyelids to prevent accidental blinking. It is best not to resist blinking. If the urge comes to you, indulge it. It will help you relax. It is my job to see that the eye in question does not blink. Meanwhile, your other eye might feel better if it is allowed to blink.

Measuring the Thickness of the Cornea

At the beginning of the surgery I will shine an unbelievably bright light into your eye for a few min-

The Surgery and How to Prepare for It

utes. It may bother you a lot at first, but this irritation will extinguish itself quickly. I will place a small probe on your cornea and take multiple readings of the corneal thickness. I use these readings to set the depth of the incision so my scalpel will not penetrate into the all important endothelial layer.

The Diamond Scalpel

The scalpel which I use in my surgery is manufactured by Coopervision-Koi. The handle of this very special scalpel is designed so that a twist in either direction will lengthen or shorten the blade. The blade extends between two small foot-like projections which actually rest on the corneal surface during the surgery and which dictate just how far into that surface the incision will be made. These feet must be highly polished so that they may glide along the surface of the cornea without tearing it.

The blade itself retracts into the handle when not in use, somewhat like the head of a turtle retracts for protection into its shell. The care of this blade is an obsession with every RK surgeon as the success of every operation depends upon the integrity of the diamond tip of this blade. Even the slightest imperfection may cause the operation to be totally ineffective. If the blade touches anything except the eye, it may be damaged beyond use. On average, I find that I am able to use one of these incredibly sharp and expensive blades only ten times before it is no longer usable. In order to be prepared for any eventuality, I keep several of these scalpels at constant readiness. Were it not for the speedy service of Federal Express, which permits me to secure repair services on one of these

I Can See!

terrifically expensive instruments on a mere two days notice, I would need to keep a great many more on hand.

The Surgical Microscope

The single most expensive piece of equipment which I use in this procedure is the operating microscope. I prefer the Wild (pronounced "Vild") microscope for a number of reasons which are purely personal, although many of my colleagues prefer the Zeiss scope.

The Wild microscope is capable of the extreme magnification necessary to allow me to adjust the length of the exposed diamond blade. This adjustment is so critical that if it is too short, the operation will not work, if it is too long, it will perforate the cornea. The margin of error in this adjustment is less than the thickness of one page of this book! I have found no other task so difficult, more taxing or requiring any greater concentration than this measurement. The hand and eye must work perfectly together to achieve the kind of accuracy which dictates the quality of performance. Every heartbeat is transmitted to the fingertips during this adjustment so that the microscope goes in and out of focus accordingly. The trick is to make the measurement between pulses! Sometimes, I think that following this step, the rest of the procedure is anticlimactic.

It is procedures like this adjustment which mean that surgeons must really have their act together, as they say, in order to accomplish this level of accuracy. Too much coffee, a hangover, domestic turmoil, or even employee dissension could make it impossible for me

The Surgery and How to Prepare for It

to deliver the tiny and precise strokes with this scalpel upon which the success of the operation depends.

The Incisions

The eye is gently but firmly grasped on two sides at its equator by a special forceps which will prevent it from turning while the central zone of the cornea is carefully and precisely marked by an optical zone marker. I have set the measurements on this ring according to the degree of the correction your visual handicap requires, figuring in such variables as age and sex. The transient impression made by pressing this circular instrument onto your cornea is centered to coincide with your point of sharpest vision. While holding your eye immobile with one hand, the surgeon's other hand makes the incisions with the scalpel.

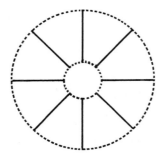

Figure 15: Diagram of the Cornea with RK Incisions.

You will not be able to see the actual incisions or instruments, just occasional glints as light is reflected onto the retina from them. The length of time which these incisions require depends upon several technical factors. However, the eye cannot remain open and exposed to air for a prolonged period of time. Were the eye to remain open too long, the corneal surface would dry and prevent the knife from gliding over it easily and the resultant damage to the epithelium, that layer covering the outside of the cornea, would be great.

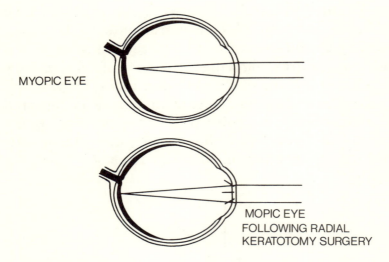

MYOPIC EYE

MOPIC EYE
FOLLOWING RADIAL
KERATOTOMY SURGERY

Figure 16: Side Views of Eye and Cornea Before RK Incisions and after RK Incisions.

The Postoperative Experience

When the incisions are completed, more drops are put into the eye, and a sterile patch is applied. This patch has no miraculous powers. I remember that immediately after my own RK surgery, I threw it away within an hour or so after I left the surgeon's office.

Patients sometimes attribute importance to such small things as this eye patch. For example, the wife of one patient, on whom I had operated the preceding

The Surgery and How to Prepare for It

Friday, called me at 2:30 Saturday morning to inquire if it were okay to remove the patches. Because he was from out-of-town, and I require all patients to come in for an examination the day after the surgery, he had checked into a motel overnight. She told me that the motel was on fire and that she needed permission to remove his patches so he could see well enough to go down the fire escape. I told you there were a lot of questions that keep recurring. If you are ever in an emergency situation such as this one, remember it is okay to remove your patches!

When you leave my office, the first thing I advise you to do is eat something. Your eye will become uncomfortable within an hour, and the pain medication may make you sick if you take it on an empty stomach. This period is where you pay your dues, as they say. The next three days will be best endured by getting as much sleep as possible because keeping your eyes closed during this period is the best thing you can do for yourself. I do not prescribe narcotic pain medications after the first night, because I suspect that they alter the internal pressure of the eye. Anything which does this could decrease the effect of the surgery.

AVOID THE USE OF MARIJUANA ABSOLUTELY DURING THE FIRST THREE WEEKS FOLLOWING RK SURGERY

The use of marijuana during the first three weeks following RK surgery will very likely result in the regression of the correction to the extent that there may be no improvement whatsoever.

I cannot say this too often or too strongly. Avoiding the use of cannabis sativa in all its varieties and preparations is an absolute necessity during this time. You would be amazed at the number of patients who will deny the use of marijuana before the surgery, and who continue to use it over my express prohibitions afterwards. Three months later when these individuals return for re-operation, my examination of the eye shows that there has been significant undercorrection of vision. Yet my examination provides no reason why this should be so. The incisions are deep, their length is correct. Then I play hardball. I will say something like this: "In the interests of your future vision, would you now undergo a urine test for drugs, so I will know what to do for you?" Bingo! That brings out a full confession every time.

Please! If you are dependent upon marijuana, and have to use cannabis in any of its forms please do not have RK surgery until you have resolved your substance abuse.

The Morning After

When you awaken the following morning, remove your patches and use your eyedrops. Many times my patients report the next morning that their eyes are very sensitive to light, though some patients have very little trouble of this kind. Some patients are unable to hold their eyes open for more than two seconds at a time. Whatever your experience otherwise, you will probably notice a distinct improvement in your vision. The miracle that is RK has already begun. Dark sunglasses may be necessary for most of the following week. Your eyes may water for several days, but you will be unable to wipe them because touching the eyelids can be very painful. Remember, this is completely normal, and part of the expected postoperative experience. It is okay to take a shower and wash your hair, just be careful when drying your face around the eyes. Vision may fluctuate widely and rapidly during the first two or three days, even changing between heartbeats. This, too, is normal.

YOUR EYES MAY BE VERY SENSITIVE TO LIGHT AFTER THE SURGERY.

The First Check-up

Normally, I try to see each patient the day after surgery, so you will have an appointment you must not miss. Do not try to drive. You must wait until you are certain you can see well enough to handle the daylight before you try to drive a car. The effects of sedation may distort your reaction time behind the wheel, so it is obvious that you should give yourself plenty of time to recover fully from the sedative effects of your medication before attempting to drive.

This visit on the day following your surgery is indispensable if brief. The primary function of this visit is to check for the initial stages of infection. As infection is the greatest risk of the postoperative period, it is crucial that you permit the surgeon to conduct an examination, to provide you with detailed instructions which will enable you to care for yourself properly and to set a date for your next visit. One of the most remarkable things you will notice on this visit is how wondrous is the change in your visual ability. It will probably take you at least a year to break the habit of reaching for your glasses, or trying to reposition them

I Can See!

on your nose. But if you are like most of my patients,
you will find this only reminds you once more of the
extraordinary transformation you have undergone.

> A SIGNIFICANT NUMBER OF PATIENTS BE-
> COME TEMPORARILY FARSIGHTED AFTER
> SURGERY, MAKING IT DIFFICULT FOR
> THEM TO DO A GREAT DEAL OF CLOSE-UP
> WORK FOR SOME TIME THEREAFTER.

*The Phenomenon of Personality Change Occasioned by
RK*

The period after surgery is one of the most reward-
ing for me. I have been astonished to witness patients
who were previously shy and reticent become outgoing
and self-confident individuals whose world is no
longer confined by the perceptual handicap that so
long oppressed them. If you follow the pattern of most
of my patients, then you too will discover a greater
feeling of self-worth in the three months following the
surgery. Though I have not found any research in the
literature to confirm my suspicions, I have come to
believe that this phenomenon of personality transformation which I observe in my patients is often the
result of an emotional weakness caused by the perceptual weakness.

When the perceptual weakness is corrected, the
root cause of the emotional weakness is removed. Individuals who have never experienced the trauma of
myopia cannot quite comprehend how this might be
possible. However, the more we learn about the deep
interconnectedness of perception and the nature of

consciousness, the more clear the presence of this emotional involvement becomes.

The First Week After the Operation

During the first week after RK surgery, ten percent of my patients notice that reading is difficult, if not impossible, and that their distance vision is not so great either. This realization usually appears like clockwork during the fourth day following the surgery and will doubtless provoke them to call their surgeon's office. No matter how prepared they might be for this event, it nearly always comes as something of a shock. This temporary farsightedness is most likely caused by the swelling of the cornea, and may last for three days to a month or longer.

DURING STABILIZATION, IT IS VERY COMMON TO EXPERIENCE FLUCTUATION OF VISION FROM DAY TO DAY AND FROM MORNING TO NIGHT.

Older patients have sometimes found this condition lasts for up to three months. Some patients discover it is very annoying to have to wear glasses even though before the operation they could read quite well without glasses. Ironically, on more occasions than not this condition is a very good sign, as it seems to predict that the surgery will be successful. This temporary condition is most easily corrected by wearing reading glasses which are inexpensive and can be purchased at a drugstore. Such glasses are available in a range of powers, and you should look for a plus sign with a numerical designation following, such as"+2.50." The higher the number, the more powerful the glasses.

Immediate Side Effects of the Surgery

After about two weeks, sensitivity to light usually diminishes greatly, although many patients may still experience a little glare. This kind of glare is comparable to that which contact lens wearers experience. If the eyes were sensitive to light before the operation, they will remain so afterward. Sometimes when observing bright lights after dark—perhaps when they see the headlights of an oncoming car—a few of my patients experience this glare as a "starburst." Even this kind of starburst glare will become less pronounced with time, although theoretically it could be permanent.

> A LARGE PERCENTAGE OF RK PATIENTS EXPERIENCE A TEMPORARY STARBURST EFFECT WHEN LOOKING AT LIGHTS. SOME CASES HAVE BEEN PERMANENT.

The eyes may be quite red for five or six days after the surgery. This condition will resolve itself with a little time. This redness is a normal side effect of the manipulation of the tissues of the eye which are part of the surgery and is not an indication of infection. It usually happens that one eye feels better than the other during recovery. Remember that they are both supposed to feel irritated. So you should regard this as a half-blessing rather than a half-curse. In addition, the eyes may water profusely at times for up to ten days to three weeks after the surgery. This also is a completely expected reaction and should not be alarming.

SIGNIFICANT CHANGES IN VISION COULD OCCUR FOR THREE OR MORE MONTHS AFTER SURGERY.

You should be alarmed, however, if after twenty-four hours or so following the operation, you notice that your eyes are producing a very yellow and quite thick secretion or pus. This yellow secretion will collect and must be wiped away every sixty seconds or so. The eye can produce considerable quantities of this fluid when it is attacked by certain bacteria. I have never observed this in any of my surgical patients, although I have seen it in wearers of soft contact lenses especially of the extended- wear variety, so it is not impossible.

Matted eyelashes, crusted eyelids, and stickiness are not signs of serious infection. They only signify the production of mucus, which can be quite pronounced at times.

However, it is never produced in the extreme quantities which occasions serious infection where frank pus is produced.

Should you notice the presence of such a pus, you must not delay in seeking medical attention.

I Can See!

The Second Surgery

If at the end of three months your vision remains good, then you can cautiously celebrate. As I have said earlier, I designed this procedure so that there is a tendency to require two surgeries to minimize the possibility of over correction. Many patients will discover that this means that they do not need the second stage, as their disability is fully corrected as a result of the first surgery. For those who do need further correction, glasses may have to be worn prior to the second surgery. I usually recommend that if a patient's daytime vision is close to 20/20, that the second surgery be delayed for several months, as small improvements sometimes occur during this time. I find that many people are very impatient during this period and seem willing to take far more risks with their eyesight than I can allow.

> REPEAT SURGERY MAY BE PERFORMED ONLY IF YOUR PHYSICIAN DEEMS IT TO BE APPROPRIATE.

Remember, your RK surgeon has a vastly larger experience base on which to judge these risks, so don't try to get him to re-operate before he thinks it is advisable.

Visual Epiphanies Which Result from RK Surgery

I continue to be amazed by the small epiphanies my patients share with me when they can finally see without their glasses. Sometimes when people go shopping for the first time without their eyeglasses, they discover that they must relearn the correct size of objects. Wearing glasses to correct nearsightedness causes things to look smaller and even contacts do this to a lesser degree. On more than one occasion since my RK surgery, I have purchased what I thought was the correct size of frozen juice, only to discover upon returning home that my pitcher was too small to hold the diluted product. Your improved peripheral vision will contain other surprises. If you wore glasses previously, you will discover that where the rims of your glasses once were, now whole fields of activity and color exist. Now you won't have to turn your head to see to the side. And your friends will continually be surprised at how different you look, how much younger you seem, forgetting all the while that for all those years you wore glasses.

7

The RK Controversy

The Long History of Scientific Controversy
If the history of science teaches us anything, it teaches us that nothing of any scientific value ever enters the cultural and social mainstream without an accompanying controversy. We do not have to look too closely at the history of those things most of us consider an essential part of our daily lives to discover the brouhaha which occasioned their appearance.

The controversy over many scientific technologies and concepts still rings in our ears. No less a man than Galileo was forced by the Church to recant his discovery that the earth circled the sun and was not—as was then thought—at the center of the universe. As one of the legends surrounding the man who first brought printing with moveable type to Europe has it, when Gutenberg first took his printed bibles to Paris where no two books had ever been virtually identical before, he was almost burned at the stake as a witch. In order to save himself, the story goes, he had to reveal important trade secrets.

I Can See!

Even daylight saving time did not find and has not found universal acceptance without opposition.

So perhaps we should not be surprised that when a Russian physician asserts he has invented a surgical procedure which will replace glasses and contact lenses, there is a certain amount of controversy in response. Furthermore, when this surgery goes on a revolutionary assembly line footing in the Soviet Union, it is perhaps understandable that Western surgeons should be hesitant and cautious.

RK, at this stage in its history, is controversial. It is controversial in the same way that contact lenses or coronary bypass surgery were controversial in the beginning. In this chapter I wish to explore with you very candidly my understanding of the reasons why radial keratotomy is controversial. In doing this we will discuss those groups who generally oppose radial keratotomy and what their reasons for opposing radial keratotomy have been, in my opinion.

Who Regulates RK? Not the FDA!

In our society we have worked very diligently to regulate the pharmaceutical industry and to impose rigorous licensing procedures upon physicians and surgeons so that the public would be protected from the abuses which so often afflicted the populace in the nineteenth century. The pharmaceutical industry is regulated by the Food and Drug Administration (FDA) which demands very high levels of testing and validification of effects before a drug enters the American marketplace. We should recall perhaps the controversy over the FDA's refusal to license the drug, thalidomide, for distribution in this country, despite its widespread acceptance as a remedy for insomnia in foreign countries. The FDA's decision was primarily influenced by one official who feared that the drug might not be safe for the unborn children of women who were pregnant when they used the drug.

The furor leveled at this official was enormous, and most of it seemed justified at the time. Accusations of capriciousness were common, but this official stood her ground. While the FDA conducted preliminary testing on a limited basis to determine its safety, in those countries where the drug was readily prescribed deformed infants began to be delivered with increasing frequency to women who had taken thalidomide. When it suddenly became obvious that the FDA had been correct, the criticism died abruptly. Many individuals in the generation born during the early sixties when this controversy raged owe the soundness of their bodies to the courageous intransigence of this one official.

There is another side to this regulatory process. In this case, there are many deserving drugs which as a result of this regulatory process have been unnecessarily withheld from the market. It now takes many years for a new drug to reach patients. Consequently, when one drug does secure approval, its retail cost must reflect not only the extensive testing required to reach the public, but the research costs of the hundreds of other drugs which did not secure such approval. It is no wonder that generic drugs are less expensive. By the time a drug has become available in generic form, most of the research costs have been recovered. It is very likely that under today's regulatory environment, neither aspirin nor penicillin would have been allowed to come to market, such are the potentially adverse effects inherent in each drug.

On the other hand, our society has not found the need to regulate innovative surgical procedures in the same way. The FDA is not given that responsibility. I am often asked by my patients, "Does this operation have FDA approval?" It is very difficult to explain to most people that unless a device such as a pacemaker or some other manufactured product is incorporated into the surgery, the operation is not regulated by any government authority. There is no agency of the Federal Government or State Government which has the authority to regulate any medical procedure that does not implant a device into the body of the patient or involve radical new technology.

How Do We Know When an Operation Is Safe?

As I have tried to establish on more than one occasion in this book, medicine is not an exact science. It is not as easy to "test" a surgical procedure as it is to test a highly machined device, or carefully researched drug. Unlike the so called "hard sciences" in which exact replication of an experimental result is essential, modern medicine is based upon statistical evidence. Because the human body is such a complex and astonishingly intricate system, the number of variables that come into play in medical results is beyond our ability to articulate and account for. Consequently, physicians must look at the long range effect of a surgical procedure upon a large body of individuals and establish trends. For example, until recently it was thought that everyone who had abdominal surgery should have the appendix removed in the same operation, to avoid possible bouts of appendicitis in the future. This is rarely practiced now, as the appendix may have some small role in contributing to the body's immunological resistance to cancer.

Moreover, some branches of medicine have been demonstrated to have a higher degree of accuracy in diagnosis prior to surgery than others. Two such branches are urology and ophthalmology. Unlike a urological surgical procedure, however, the results of ophthalmological surgery are very evident almost from the first moment of recovery. A patient recovering from RK, for example, will know the outcome of his operation before anyone else: he cannot be deceived, because he can see the result for himself. In my thinking, the opinions of RK patients must be given a great deal of weight but at the same time such testimonials must be balanced by statistical evidence and case histories.

Who Regulates RK?
The Ruling of the Academy of Ophthalmology:
"Investigational Status"

The accepted opinion of medical experts is that no patient is qualified to evaluate any operation. Consequently, we are forced to turn to the collective wisdom of the physicians who most frequently deal with the operation and its results. In the case of ophthalmology that organization is the American Academy of Ophthalmology. It was the work of the predecessors of this group of physicians which took the very first steps towards board certification of physicians specializing in the diseases and defects of the eye. Indeed, the first board examinations for any branch of medicine were administered to ophthalmologists in Memphis, Tennessee, before World War I.

The Academy holds a high level of concern for the welfare of all patients, and great censure is brought to bear on any doctor who performs "unnecessary surgery." As you might expect, the approval of this body for any new procedure is very difficult to obtain. Most of the members of the American Academy of Ophthalmology who must make decisions regarding policies probably wish that RK had never been invented. Here is an operation which from all evidence seems to work very well, but is relatively recent in its origin. Like the FDA, the American Academy of Ophthalmology is very conservative in its judgments and realizes that it will not be embarrassed if it waits for years before declaring the surgery "approved." On the other hand, cases like that of the FDA's reluctance to give its approval to thalidomide, are ample demonstration that speedy approval can on occasion be embarrassing. Obviously, the justification for the refusal to rush to judgement is that if a responsible medical organization publicly designates a procedure safe and that procedure later is found to be suspect, then it risks public disrepute, and professional abandonment. Far better to let time and the profession prove the procedure before the official seal of approval goes on.

Regulatory agencies usually have three levels of acceptance through which drugs and medical devices must pass: "Experimental," "Investigational," and "Approved." The rating "Experimental" means that the product is so new that no judgment has been made on its value. "Investigational" indicates that the product has shown considerable merit, and sufficient demonstration of safety in animals has been shown to warrant exposure of human subjects to the product, under strict controls. The designation "Approved" indicates that a product has been found to be safe and effective for general use.

Operations are not regulated on a procedure-by-procedure basis in the same way that drugs and medical devices are because surgeons go through a fiercely rigorous credentialing process as part of their training and licensing, and because a surgical procedure is not as quantifiable as a chemical formula or a mechanical blueprint. In many cases, the craft and art of the surgeon is as important as the theoretical and anatomical aspects of any surgical procedure. Hence the medical profession has always credentialed, and the state has always licensed, the individual rather than the procedure.

Even so, the American Medical Association and the professional associations of medical specialists such as the American Academy of Ophthalmology have established the practice of following regulatory agencies by designating surgical procedures as "Experimental," "Investigational," or "Approved" *even though they have no legal regulatory power whatsoever to enforce their designations.* The medical profession has seen many surgical procedures remain in the investigational stage for years while surgeons perform them upon literally thousands of patients. That is to say, that an operation receives the approval status tacitly long before any responsible organization publicly confirms it. The American Medical Association follows the lead of the American Academy of Ophthalmology in designating this procedure "Investigational."

111

I Can See!

One of the main points contained in the policy statement of the American Academy of Ophthalmology regarding RK which has not been revised since 1985, focuses on the possibility of long-term damage, which has not been sufficiently assessed (See Appendix A). As an RK surgeon, I have been puzzled by this policy statement. On the one hand, the Academy seems to be saying, "We do not have to make up our minds on this procedure yet, and in order to evaluate the long term implications of RK we must wait for many years." On the other, it seems to be an easy way to avoid making a hard decision, especially a decision which affects only a small minority of its members. The percentage of opthalmologists who regularly perform RK is less than ten. While the Academy has withheld its approval of the procedure, it is interesting to note that during each annual convention it spends a great deal of time and money teaching the techniques of RK surgery to its members. These courses are both well taught and well attended.

In contrast to the Academy's position on RK is the general position on the implantation of intraocular lenses. According to this policy it is permissible to implant an intraocular lens into a cataract patient who may be only twenty-two years of age. As a matter of policy this is not frowned upon, though some ophthalmologists object to it strenuously. In fact, cataract surgery destroys about ten percent of the precious endothelial cells lining the inside of the human cornea. The implantation of the intraocular lens destroys another eight percent. When this surgical destruction of the irreplaceable endothelial layer of the cornea is compounded by the natural deterioration of this layer

112

due to the ageing process we can see that the potential long term damage to the endothelial function may reach the point that the cornea will not be able to maintain its transparency, and blindness may be the result. Admittedly, this is a worst-case scenario and not typical of the average cataract patient. Even so, this result has occurred many times. As opthalmologists we are able to approve such a risk in intraocular lens implantation because without the procedure the patient would be blind in that eye. Assuredly, such is not the case with RK, but I am forced to wonder if the fact that the number of surgeons who perform this implantation surgery is greater than that who perform RK is not of equal importance. Perhaps my cynicism is showing but, as the Academy of Ophthalmology is an organization of physicians who are also human, it is logical to suspect the numerical bias to be significant.

As a surgeon who has undertaken both intraocular lens implantation and radial keratotomy in a large enough volume to be able to speak with some authority on both subjects, I can tell you that cataract surgery, while highly technical and sophisticated, requires only a fraction of the attention to detail that RK demands. Specifically, RK requires a mechanical device to measure the thickness of the cornea to within 0.025 millimeters, an absolutely flawless diamond scalpel capable of delivering an exact cut, as well as the skill to handle the scalpel to cut through ninety percent of that corneal thickness. For this reason a surgeon who is successful at cataract surgery may not be as successful at RK surgery. Our numbers may continue to be fewer as a result, and if there may be said to be a political agenda in this designation of RK as "Investigational" then it is unlikely that the numerical equation will shift markedly.

Regulation by Referral of Patients from Other Physicians

Few professions operate by what some have derisively called the "good old boy network" as intensively as the medical profession. Who you know and the status of your professional reputation is very important in securing patients by referral from other physicians. For decades our profession has been largely self regulating by this means. When the AMA lifted the longstanding policy and advertising for patients was deemed no longer unethical, some of this potential for self regulation was reduced. The realization that the "good old boy network," which had for so long dominated the profession, might not be in the best interest of the profession was long in coming. Perhaps the most telling force at work in the medical marketplace which forced this issue was the privatization of hospitals and the burgeoning for-profit medical industry. As a result, the number of physicians advertising their medical services has exploded. RK surgeons find that the bad press RK has unfairly received during the 80's requires them to advertise their services more extensively than some other specialties.

The controversy among ophthalmologists over the efficacy of RK has diminished referrals as a source of patients. Now I would never accuse one surgeon of being jealous of another, but of all the medical professions few specialties are given the recognition, the pressure of competition, and the media access that surgeons have gained. It is not unreasonable to admit that we are more likely to experience what has been called in other professions, the "prima donna" syndrome. But if ever there were a situation more likely to be tainted by one of those proverbial "sour grapes" attitudes, it is manifested by those ophthalmologists who have tried RK surgery, only to abandon it for "lack of effectiveness."

The Apparent Regulation of RK By Insurance Organizations

The American Medical Association and the Academy of Ophthalmology are the most widely used professional sources of ratings for any surgical procedure. Who uses such ratings? Insurance companies make considerable use of these ratings to determine which surgical expenses they should bear and which they should not. Those who do not want to bear the expense of RK surgery will quote the ratings of these two organizations in their evaluations offered in explanation of why they will not cover RK. Uninformed patients fall for this on the assumption that the American Medical Association and the Academy of Ophthalmology, like the FDA, have the legal regulatory authority to make such ratings as valid as those of the FDA. Of course, as we have seen, this is not the case.

One patient called me after receiving a letter from Blue Cross informing him that they would not reimburse him for his RK surgery. He wanted to know why Blue Cross would pay for a sex change operation but not for RK surgery. His was a good question. He decided to go ahead with the surgery, threatening to bring suit against Blue Cross for non-coverage of RK

I Can See!

surgery. I was quite surprised some time later when I received a check from Blue Cross paying the full amount for his operation. I made a photocopy of this check and hung it on the wall in my office, much as a big game hunter might display a trophy-quality rhino's head.

The Military Prohibition of RK Surgery

The military establishment has taken the absolute position that any applicant who has had RK surgery may not become a member of our armed forces. In contrast, the inductees of all Soviet military branches are given RK surgery, if they are near-sighted.

> THE ARMED SERVICES STRONGLY DIS-COURAGES MILITARY PERSONNEL AGAINST RADIAL KERATOTOMY. HAVING THE SURGERY COULD DISQUALIFY THE PATIENT FROM MILITARY SERVICE.

If this surgery is as dangerous as many say it is, then we should reduce our military spending dramatically, because if we ever square off against the Soviets, we won't need expensive weapons to defeat an army composed largely of blind soldiers! Sound silly? Of course it is. But if RK is as valuable as many of us who have had the surgery think it is, then as we begin to rely increasingly upon conventional warfare we may be facing a military cadre less dependent upon soft contact lenses which require a relatively hygienic environment to be effective and glasses, which are relatively fragile.

Actually, I have undertaken RK on military personnel, and none have ever been dismissed from the services to my knowledge, despite the government's admonition that the RK constitutes tampering with government property, thus rendering a patient vulnerable to court-martial. On the other hand, I have never gotten one of my patients into the air as a military pilot. No matter how many letters I write to Senators, Representatives, the Surgeon General, or even the President of the United States on their behalf, none has ever been forgiven an RK transgression. Apparently the military has been able to spot them through a detailed ophthalmological examination which is not given routinely to any other group of military personnel.

I do not deny that there is a potential problem in letting soldiers have RK. I have worked extensively throughout my career in Veteran's Administration hospitals, and I have seen the abuse of the system by which some few individuals have sought to gain medical disabilities far beyond their actual injuries. That these few jeopardized the benefits justly deserved by many of our valiant servicemen is a disaster of major proportions. But given the potential in our legal system for these few to generate massive litigations, the wisdom of not following the Soviet model may be peculiar to our democratic system and not related to the value of the surgery itself.

The Role of Hospitals in Regulating Access to RK

When eye surgeons admitted patients to hospitals for week-long stays associated with cataract surgery, it was fairly easy to convince hospital administrators to purchase the expensive equipment necessary to perform our most sophisticated cataract procedures. Then it occurred to some of us to question the need for the long hospital stay. Shortly thereafter, it occurred to Medicare to question the need for the long hospital stay. It did not take the industry long to realize that these operations could be undertaken effectively in ambulatory surgical centers which would cause patients less emotional trauma by returning them swiftly to their families for recuperation. Most cataract patients are elderly and, given the American medical system, they know the probability is very high that some day they will enter a hospital and not leave alive. As a consequence of this fear, most cataract patients welcome the opportunity to have their surgery in a non-hospital context.

As a consequence of this trend in the industry, hospital administrators have become reluctant to invest in surgical microscopes and other expensive cataract surgery equipment. Getting them to purchase the highly technical equipment necessary to do RK surgery is nearly impossible since they recognize that the return on their investment is likely to be low. Further, as we have seen, not all ophthalmologists are also RK surgeons, consequently it is likely that the RK surgeons on a hospital Ophthalmology staff will be in a distinct minority. Few hospitals will invest in expensive equipment which would be used by such a small number of surgeons.

As a result of these industry trends, the start-up costs associated with RK surgery fall heavily on the individual surgeon. If hospitals will not support the surgery by investing in the expensive equipment then the financial risk the RK surgeon accepts is potentially enormous. Not only will this RK surgeon need to equip his own ambulatory surgical center, but he must also be confident in his own skill and in the value of the surgery to believe the risk worthwhile. This increased financial risk not only means that even fewer ophthalmologists will become RK surgeons, but also that if they accept the risk then RK must become for them not just one procedure of many offered to their patients, but that it must be a central service that may ultimately become the focus of their practices.

THE MAJOR COMPLAINTS OF THE INDUSTRY:
Inaccuracy

Now that we have seen the way in which the medical industry certifies RK surgeons and advises the public on the status of the surgery, we should look at the three complaints which are most often heard when a prospective patient encounters the controversy surrounding the value of RK. The first of these complaints is that it is an inaccurate procedure.

WHILE SOME CASES DO REGRESS, IT IS EXTREMELY RARE FOR ANYONE'S EYES TO RETURN TO BEING AS NEARSIGHTED AS THEY WERE BEFORE THE SURGERY.

By "inaccuracy" critics of the procedure mean it is difficult to predict the degree of correction to the unaided focal length which the surgery will bring. As long as surgeons are dealing with human tissue and a healing process which is influenced by a patient's diet and metabolism, and not glass or plastic lenses there will be some validity in this criticism. Human tissue is always going to be less predictable than machined materials.

I have already dealt with the biology behind this complaint in some detail in Chapter Three, but it is important to amplify this discussion here. In my own practice I have found the correction in RK to be far more predictable than that correction available through the implantation of intraocular lenses in cataract surgery. Of course, the nature of the complaint which dictates that one patient may need RK rather than lens implantation is very different. However, that being said, I can observe that most patients who have had implantation surgery must wear glasses for distant vision, while the great majority of RK patients do not.

One class of patients on whom I perform RK will always need glasses. These are patients whose myopia is so severe prior to the operation that the surgery can never correct their vision to the degree that they can be freed from wearing glasses. They are not good candidates for RK, and I regularly advise them that RK is not going to liberate them from glasses. For some reason, I let them convince me that they would rather wear glasses with thinner lenses and that they are willing to accept this as the predictable correction RK will bring them. Even though these patients regularly sign a statement admitting that they understand RK will not bring them 20/20 vision before surgery, many will later tell me they expected to have good crisp vision after RK. Somehow they were looking for a miracle, and while RK is often called miraculous by patients with less severe myopia, there are real limits to what can be achieved for these patients. In my practice as it currently is constituted such patients represent fifteen percent of all my surgical procedures. I would like to reduce this kind of patient to less than one percent, but I have had difficulty in turning such pleas for help aside.

> AFTER THE SURGERY THE MAJORITY OF RK PATIENTS SEE WELL ENOUGH THAT THEY DO NOT WEAR ANY CORRECTIVE LENSES.

If we omit this group of patients, then the rest of the population of myopes who come to me for RK surgery fall within the range of effectiveness for this operation, and in most cases will have the potential of achieving 20/20 vision without glasses. Of these, one percent are under-responders. For these under-responders the surgery will have less than its predicted effect, and they will still need glasses. No matter how many times they have the surgery they will not achieve full correction. These people apparently have an unusual ability to heal their corneal wounds by linking the corneal fibers across the RK incisions in such a way that most of the effect is negated. Various measures have been tried to help these patients achieve better results, but none have been satisfactory. I have had ten such patients in my practice as of this writing and each of them is waiting to see what the new research in this field might offer them. There is hope for these patients on the horizon which I will describe in a later chapter.

For the remainder of patients within the normal range of effectiveness, fully ninety-nine percent will be able to drive without their eyeglasses. This implies a visual acuity of 20/30 or better. A high percentage of these patients are able to perform all tasks without glasses. Ninety percent of them achieve 20/20 vision. Many of them require two operations on each eye to achieve this, but this is true only because I am very conservative in the way I structure my surgical procedure so as to minimize the risk of overcorrection. Remember that overcorrection has been the bane of this procedure in the national experience.

Of course, patients over forty years of age may have to wear glasses to read, but this is a normal function of the ageing process and as I have tried to emphasize RK is not a remedy for the effects of middle and old age.

> IT MAY TAKE SEVERAL DAYS FOR NORMAL VISUAL ACUITY TO BE ACHIEVED AFTER RK. IN SOME CASES, UP TO SIX MONTHS HAVE BEEN NECESSARY FOR STABILIZATION OF VISION.

THE MAJOR COMPLAINTS OF THE INDUSTRY:
RK Is a Cosmetic Procedure

One of the most frequently heard objections to RK, especially from the insurance industry as one company or another tries to explain why they do not cover this surgery, is that it is a cosmetic procedure. In my opinion this is utter nonsense. In the first place, the condition of myopia is not disfiguring, and in the second place the effects of RK are invisible to the naked eye. How then can this be considered cosmetic surgery, one might ask? The obvious response is that it rids the patient of the need to wear glasses. Are we to assume then that glasses are disfiguring? Surely optometrists would object to this notion.

Quite the opposite is often true. Many people believe that wearing glasses is quite stylish, and some young executives wear glasses with window glass lenses in order to look older. Specialists in the "dress for success" field sometimes even advise such glasses as props to use in the office, so they can tweak their chin with the earpieces to appear contemplative, or slam them down on the desk when emphasis is needed in a negotiation.

Well, perhaps, RK is cosmetic because it rids the RK patient of the need to wear contacts? But are contacts disfiguring? Surely not. Inconvenient perhaps. Even on occasion contacts may become a source of possible visual impairment or damage.

The use of RK to eliminate contacts may in fact be enlightened rather than cosmetic. If we shift sensory organs for a minute, we will see how peculiar this argument really is. If you are hard of hearing and eliminate an unsightly hearing-aid, then according to current insurance company practices that is not cosmetic surgery, it is beneficial and necessary surgery. So surgical correction of hearing is not cosmetic but the surgical correction of vision is? What an interesting world we live in.

I Can See!

So how do you explain such a clear logical contra-diction? The population of the hearing impaired is somewhat smaller (twenty million) than the propor-tion of the population which is visually impaired. Fur-thermore, there is considerably more sympathy for wearers of hearing aids than for those who wear glasses. My sometimes cynical self wonders what rhetoric insurance companies would use to defend their refusal to cover this surgery, if more of the popu-lation became hearing impaired and this surgical pro-cedure for hearing became more popular.

Now, I hasten to add that truly deaf people have a hard time in this world, and I have long felt that we need a concerted effort to sensitize the general public to comprehend the sense of isolation these hearing im-paired individuals experience. But the hearing im-paired are no less isolated than the visually impaired. The logic of this discrimination seems based more upon the numerical size of the visually impaired popu-lation who might want RK and the impact which such a population might have upon the financial reserves of the insurance industry should RK become as popular as it promises to become.

In my opinion, RK patients suffer an unusual dis-crimination from insurance companies for no reason other than an economic one. In short, if any organ of the human body can be made to function more nor-mally by surgery then it follows that any individual possessing such a dysfunctional organ should be al-lowed to receive such surgery without the use of such an illogical argument as this one most surely is, when the speciousness of that argument fools no one.
(See Appendix B).

124

The RK Controversy

THE MAJOR COMPLAINTS OF THE INDUSTRY:
RK Is an Unnecessary Procedure

The last objection I wish to deal with, one my patients often tell me they have heard, is that RK is unnecessary. Is RK necessary? Well in the sense that RK is not correcting a life threatening medical condition, it is not necessary. In the sense that RK is not correcting a condition which left untreated would cause blindness, it is not necessary. But see here, if such logic was applied uniformly throughout the medical industry, this rationale might have some merit. Of course, it seems to be applied only when an insurance company finds it convenient to avoid exposing itself to a significant economic liability.

For example, many cardiologists consider cardiac bypass surgery to be unnecessary, but it is denied to no one who has evidence of coronary artery obstruction, and the insurance companies do not refuse to cover the procedure. Surgery for patients with most lung cancers is unnecessary, since these patients usually die anyway. As it is thought less unpleasant to die from the spreading of cancer to other vital organs, than from the lesions in the lung itself, no one is denied such surgery, and the insurance companies do not fail to cover the procedure.

Abortions are seldom necessary to preserve the life of the expectant mother, but few who find it inconvenient to be pregnant are denied an abortion. Insurance companies receive a positive economic benefit if a mother chooses to have an abortion because an abortion is far less expensive than normal childbirth, the hospitalization of two patients, plus the potential expense of benefits to be paid if either mother or child experiences complications. As a physician I have been constantly amazed by the inequities in our insurance system, and the smokescreen which each company tries to create in order to conceal the economic logic which creates them. In my experience, the dividing line between "necessary" and "convenient," like that between "necessary" and "preferred," are fine lines which always seem to be drawn for economic reasons rather than medical.

The Economic Interests of Optometrists Seem to Provoke the RK Controversy

They used to say in politics that no one can be blamed for voting their own interests. And in this way, we cannot blame optometrists if they vote their own interests in the arena of RK politics. Mind you we don't have to like it, but it is to be expected.

Myopes, as a rule, see their optometrists far more often than they see an ophthalmologist. They tend to see an ophthalmologist when they are in serious trouble and fear their vision is being compromised seriously. Consequently, the general public places a lot of faith in optometrists and opticians.

Now I hasten to say that optometrists and opticians have made an enormous contribution to the field of eye care, and by and large are as professional a group of individuals as one will find in the medical industry. However, if you could be one of those proverbial "bugs on the wall" and listen to what my patients tell me they have been told about RK by their optometrists and opticians it would make your antennae curl. Given the potential distortion in second hand testimony, I can dismiss a lot I hear in this way, but the testimony of my patients is so consistent that I must feel some amazement at the level of misinformation generated from these sources. The bottom line always seems to be that "you might go blind if you have RK." Often the prophecy includes such lines as: "You are going to have permanent scars"; or "You will have recurrent eye infections"; or "You will have trouble driving at night"; or "You will have adhesions from the scars." Unfortunately, as patients continue to explore RK and discover that they have been seriously misled, they are no longer able to trust these health care professionals. This outcome is so predictable that I am forced to wonder if the preservation of the eyeglass and contact lens franchise is worth the denigration of their reputations as health care professionals which surely is the inevitable result of such poor advice. On the other hand were it not so damaging, I would do well to consider such advice as a backhand compliment to RK inasmuch as it is in recognition of the potential inherent in RK to eliminate or greatly reduce the need for their services that the campaign of misinformation is generated.

Economic Interests of Employers Seem to Provoke the RK Controversy

Any surgical procedure such as RK is occasioned by the need to take a sick leave for recuperation. And in such time off from the job, employers for a time lose the services of their myopic employees who may be highly placed and highly valued. This is not inexpensive. Consequently, many of my patients bring to me notices formerly tacked to their bulletin boards containing tales of horror strong enough to make a grown

I Can See!

man or woman quail at the thought of eye surgery. I have heard stories of company-wide required meetings in which RK was strongly denounced by the company nurse or some visiting dignitary. Most workers are clever enough to see through the logic of such meetings and are seldom deterred from investigating the surgery further. In most cases, such meetings do little more than stimulate interest in the procedure and in the final analysis only become a source of friction between the employer and employee. The time lost in this way is minimal, but I have been amazed by patients who use up all their accrued sick leave regardless of the real time needed to recuperate from RK.

The RK Controversy Does Not Seem Likely to Go Away Any Time Soon

My goal in this chapter has been to try to expose the hidden agenda behind most sources of the controversy. Similarly, I would be amiss if I did not admit that as an RK surgeon I am biased in favor of the surgery. And I will never be able to fully convince you that my biases are based less on economic goals than on the desire to offer a remedy for myopia to individuals who would like to have normally functioning eyes.

As you read my apologia for RK, I hope you will see it as a balanced statement somewhere between the positions of the hostile opponents of the surgery and that of the zealots who have had the surgery and think every one should rush right out and have it.

Truly, the chances of your going blind from RK are about on a par with your dying in a plane crash.

I hope this comforts you somewhat, but I must admit that as I boarded the plane en route to keep my rendezvous with my RK surgeon, this statistic was doubly on my mind.

Please remember that I did not write this book to convince you to have RK. I wrote this book to counter the bad press surrounding RK and to use it as a patient education tool. Consequently, it is my hope that, on the one hand, this book will help you to understand the surgery more clearly so you can explain it to family and friends. On the other hand, I hope that this book will enable you to ask intelligent questions of your surgeon or medical advisor.

8

The Future of Radial Keratotomy

A very important consideration in deciding whether to have RK—if no emergency condition demands it—is the developmental status of the operation. If rapid advances are in the works, wisdom would indicate that you should wait to determine what will be available in a year or two. I write this remembering the story of the so-called "expert" who in 1912 wrote that "the automobile has now reached perfection to the point that no more improvements are possible." Still, RK has not changed significantly during the last three years, and I do not anticipate great improvements anytime soon.

There are other operations within the realm of refractive surgery which serve patients who are not ideal candidates for RK. These operations are as follows:

- Keratomileusis
- Epikeratophakia
- Lensectomy
- Corneal Mortar
- Inlaid Corneal Lenses
- Laser Surgery

I Can See!

Keratomileusis

Keratomileusis was pioneered by Dr. Barraquer of Bogata, Colombia, and involves the removal of a thin layer of the cornea including the visual axis. This tissue is attached to a lathe and frozen in liquid nitrogen until it is metal hard. The frozen layer of the cornea is then turned upon the surgical lathe to a predetermined specification yielding a flatter shape before it is stitched back upon the eye. This operation is most effective within the range of -3 to -10 diopters. Later research suggests that the freezing technique causes damage to the living tissue and that the accuracy of the correction is not as great as in RK. Moreover, astigmatism of a disturbing degree may be produced. [See T. I. Barraquer and others, "Results of Myopic Keratomileusis," *Journal of Refractive Surgery*, 3:3, 98-101.]

Some surgeons are developing methods of reshaping the tissue without freezing, and these reports in the medical literature are quite promising. Still the problems of inaccuracy and induced astigmatism remain. Recovery time is much longer than that occasioned by RK as sutures must remain in place between two weeks and two months, causing discomfort and redness of the eye. Few American surgeons practice this difficult procedure, as the equipment required is unusually expensive and rare. In capable hands, however, Keratomileusis may be a very useful procedure.

Epikeratophakia

Epikeratophakia is similar to corneal transplantation with a single important difference. The recipient does not lose his own corneal tissue in the process.

The Future of Radial Keratotomy

Donor corneas are obtained which, for one reason or another, are unsuitable for full-thickness cornea transplants. Prior to 1984 all such corneas were routinely discarded, but through epikeratophakia these donated tissues are now salvageable and useful in refractive surgery.

As in keratomileusis, the tissue is frozen and lathed according to a specific patient's needs. But at this stage epikeratophakia differs from keratomileusis as the cornea is then shipped in a dehydrated state to the surgeon where he or she prepares it for use by soaking it in the proper solution for a few minutes before surgery. [See P. S. Binder and others, "Combined Morphological Effects of Cryolathing and Lyophilizations on Epikeratoplasty Lenticues," *Arch. Ophthalmol.*, 104, (1986), 671-9.] During recovery the recipient's own corneal epithelium grows over the graft. Rejection of this tissue by the patient's immune system has been almost negligible. Early research on this procedure was performed by Drs. Kaufman and McDonald at the Louisiana State University Eye Center in New Orleans. The tissue for this extraordinary procedure is prepared by Allergan Medical Optics of Irvine, California, among others, and all donors are carefully screened for transmissible diseases, including AIDS, before the tissue is cleared for use.

Epikeratophakia is effective in the correction of myopia in the -6.00 and -20 diopter range. The grafts may also be used to correct farsightedness of large degree, as well as in the treatment of keratoconus, a condition in which the shape of the cornea is distorted by an extreme bulging. Epikeratophakia is also suitable as an alternative to intraocular lens implantation following cataract surgery. It shows special promise in infant cataract surgery, for which lens implantation is considered inadvisable. There are several drawbacks to epikeratophakia, however. Recovery may take a very long time, even up to two years. Additional procedures are often necessary in order to alleviate the large amounts of astigmatism caused when suturing the grafts in place. Marked over- and undercorrections occur, greatly compromising the accuracy of the surgery. Severe pain and redness of the eye may occur until the sutures are removed. Addiction to pain medication develops in a certain percentage of patients.

The beauty of the surgery lies in the reversibility of the procedure. The graft may be removed and replaced by another at almost any time. This is in direct contrast to RK, which is usually not reversible. The techniques of epikeratophakia are being improved rapidly, but much remains to be done before the accuracy of this procedure will be high enough for it to be generally acceptable. Still, for the severely visually handicapped individuals who cannot see clearly beyond one to five inches, epikeratophakia provides hope.

Lensectomy

There are a few advocates of lensectomy in the treatment of myopia greater than -10 diopters. The risks of lensectomy are quite significant, and include such things as retinal detachment, intraocular infection and hemorrhage, astigmatism, and inaccurate correction. It is my opinion that this procedure will not gain widespread acceptance because of these risks. There is no doubt that it works ninety-five percent of the time, but in my opinion the complication rate is too high, especially when those complications can be quite severe, even blinding.

Corneal Mortar

A substance is now being studied which may be placed within the incisions of RK to yield a greater correction than that achieved by the RK surgery itself. Reports published in mid-1986 suggested the possibility of corrections up to -20 diopters. The frequency of such reports has diminished greatly during the past six months, suggesting that the longer-term results may have been disappointing. It may not be possible to adequately calibrate the amount of correction in individual cases. I have great hope that positive results will be forthcoming, as I would welcome this addition to our armamentarium of treatment for high myopia.

Inlaid Corneal Lenses

Polysulfone is a plastic polymer which is optically clear and easily tolerated by the delicate tissue of the cornea and causes no significant rejection as a result of the foreign body rejection of the human immunological system. The basic principle behind inlaid corneal lenses is that a surgical plane may be created within the cornea, allowing the surgeon to slide in this lens to change curvature of the cornea.

Animal studies have demonstrated a tendency toward scarring in the visual axis which would sharply decrease acuity. Unfortunately, this inlaid corneal lens tends to interfere with the function of the endothelial layer, which maintains the cornea in the partially dehydrated state so necessary for transparency.

135

I Can See!

Consequently, the cornea experiences an edema or swelling which reduces clarity. Although research is underway to resolve this problem, I believe that it will be very difficult to overcome. [See Stephen S. Lane and others, "Polysulfone Intracorneal Lenses," *Journal of Refractive Surgery,* 1:5 (November-December 1985), 207-216.]

Some research is underway on softer materials which are similar to corneal tissue in that these materials have a similar state of hydration. This avenue of research may ultimately make it possible to achieve a homeostatic mechanism which will make inlaid corneal lenses a viable option. If scarring can be kept to a minimum, inlaid corneal lenses may be the future's answer to correcting myopia surgically. In my opinion, however, its greatest potential lies in its promise for correcting more severe myopia, and that it will never be as acceptable as RK for moderate cases of myopia.

Laser Surgery

Fully ninety percent of my patients ask me if RK is done by laser. Most are terribly disappointed when I tell them I use a mere diamond scalpel to make the incisions. Not only has the general public developed an enormous faith in lasers, which seem to represent technology in its highest form, but also a majority of my elderly patients have come to believe that cataracts can be removed by lasers. In fact, lasers cannot completely cure a primary cataract, as cataracts contain particles which must be mechanically removed from the eye by opening it surgically. To leave these materials floating around inside the eye would be dangerous indeed.

The Future of Radial Keratotomy

Lasers are used in eye surgery, and there are many different typse of lasers in medical use. For example, an argon laser is used to create intense heat within a tiny area, relying on tissue pigmentation to absorb laser light. However, in corneal surgery an argon laser could not create heat since the cornea is colorless—unless the surgeon artificially induces color into the cornea. Just such a strategy has been attempted by some surgeons who inject a dye, such as methylene blue, into the cornea. In some cases the laser treatment has been reported successful, although I know of no formal research documenting this work. However, I have seen no real demonstrated advantage to this method when compared to diamond-scalpel RK. The only advantage I can discover would be strictly a public relations value, one obtained by catering to the public's admiration for laser surgery.

There is, however, a new laser which shows enormous promise in refractive surgery. This new laser is called the "Excimer Laser." To create this laser, a mixture of elemental gases, including flourine, is excited by an electrical current. When this laser is focused on the corneal surface, tiny portions of the cornea are vaporized. Such a tool may eventually permit a surgeon to sculpt the cornea into virtually any desired shape or curvature.

Still experimental, there are many questions which have to be answered before the excimer laser can enjoy widespread use by eye surgeons. For example, consider the layer of cells which cover the outermost surface of the cornea, the epithelial cells. Now we have always considered Bowman's layer, that thin layer which lies just beneath the epithelial cells, to be of such vital function that corneal integrity would be compromised by its absence. Bowman's layer acts to anchor the epithelial cells to the cornea, thereby preventing the epithelium from being wiped away by blinking. Bowman's layer is destroyed by the excimer laser, but a new layer is formed which may be just as good. Only further experimentation will tell, but if the excimer laser is as promising as it seems to be, it may eventually permit us to eliminate eyeglasses and contacts entirely.

Even with all this promise of new developments in laser surgery, the risk of scarring in the visual axis cannot be ignored. Although that risk is small, it is not negligible. Therefore, I believe that radial keratotomy will stand as the treatment method of choice for mild to moderate myopia for many years to come.

Appendix A

RADIAL KERATOTOMY*

The American Academy of Ophthalmology receives periodic inquiries regarding the surgical procedure known as "radial keratotomy". While data on radial keratotomy are not complete, and therefore no definitive statement can be made, the Academy believes that the following statement may be of some assistance to those inquiring about this procedure.

Myopia (nearsightedness) is a "refractive error", causing blurred distance vision with an otherwise normal, healthy eye. Radial keratotomy is a surgical technique for modifying myopia by radial incisions in the cornea to flatten the corneal curvature.

On the basis of reports presently available, radial keratotomy continues to evolve as a surgical technique for modifying myopia, but it is too early to evaluate completely the incidence of post-operative complications or to draw conclusions regarding the long-time effects of the procedure. At this time, it appears from reports in the scientific literature that most individuals who have undergone radial keratotomy are pleased with the initial results. However, over the past several years, there have been reports in the scientific literature of unpredictable results and some instances of serious visual impairment, including blindness. In any assessment of radial keratotomy, the risk/benefit comparison is especially important. The procedure may reduce or eliminate the need of eyeglasses or contact lenses; but at least until more long-term data are available, this benefit must be weighed against the possibility of immediate or future impairment of sight or other complications. Not until a number of studies are completed will it be possible to state definitively the risks and benefits of radial keratotomy.

At this time, radial keratotomy is an investigational procedure for the modification of myopia which should be conducted in accordance with adequate review mechanisms and preceded by appropriate informed consent which recognizes the special nature and presently uncertain ramifications of the procedure.

Approved By: Academy Board of Directors
August 24, 1985

Reviewed and Reaffirmed:
June 22, 1986

*Reprinted by permission of The American Academy of Ophthalmology, 655 Beach Street, P.O. Box 7424, San Francisco, CA 94120-7424, (415) 561-8500.

Appendix B

Radial Keratotomy:
Cosmetic or Functional?*

The question: "Radial keratotomy surgery: cosmetic or functional?" can best be answered when the two aspects of the question are separated. The first aspect is the nature of the surgical procedure itself, and the second is the patient's motivation.

First, the nature of the surgery itself is not a matter for debate. It is purely a matter of fact and definition. This surgery does not enhance the beauty or appearance of the patient or his eye. It does not enlarge the eye, alter its color, or redefine its shape. The corneal scars are almost impossible to detect. Why then do some continue to contend that it is cosmetic, when it actually restores the proper focus to the eye? By definition, this surgery is functional surgery and not cosmetic. Until recently, optical devices have been a lifelong necessity for myopic persons. Now, refractive surgery such as radial keratotomy (RK) offers patients an opportunity to correct their vision rather than to constantly depend on glasses or contacts.

In other fields of medicine this is already a well-established principle. For instance, a patient with otosclerosis can hear with the assistance of a hearing aid. The aid successfully transmits sound to an otherwise healthy inner ear; however, surgery to relieve the otosclerosis, such as stapes mobilization, restores the function of the organ. It enables the patient to hear without any mechanical device. The inner ear itself has not been improved, but the mechanism to transmit the sound has been reestablished. It is true the patient no longer is required to wear a hearing aid, which he may have considered ugly and been self conscious about, but the purpose of the surgery is to restore hearing. It is functional, not cosmetic surgery.

Likewise, a patient requiring a brace to walk may be told corrective orthopedic surgery can restore the function of his defective limb. We all would consider the restoration of the proper function of his leg functional surgery. It is true, as a secondary advantage he is freed from an ugly brace or crutch; however, no one would agree with the statement that orthopedic surgery was cosmetic.

If it is not cosmetic for a person to have restored hearing or walk without aids, why is it not true for the visually-handicapped also?

If an RK patient's vision is restored to proper functioning, this is functional. It is not cosmetic, though getting rid of the mechanical optical device is a secondary result.

The second aspect of the question that should be considered is patient motivation. Why do people elect to have a refractive surgery? If the patient's primary concern is to improve his appearance, then, for him, the surgery is cosmetic.

From my own clinical observations, this has not often been the case. The vast majority of my contact lens patients definitely do indicate the primary purpose of contact lenses is cosmetic. Other considerations, such as improved peripheral vision and the ability to move their eyes without running into the restriction of the frame is less important. In sharp contrast, almost all RK patients come to my office seeking improved function. After surgery, they expressed extreme satisfaction with being able to function without dependency on optical appliances. Many patients had a better appearance with glasses than without them. Since their goal was not cosmetic, their enthusiasm following successful surgery is not a result of merely discarding glasses.

Again, patients who had been successfully wearing contact lenses before radial keratotomy obviously did not gain any measure of improved appearance. Only the small group of patients unable to wear contact lenses could be said to have gained any cosmetic advantage. However, they too stated the greatest advantage was the freedom to see any time and at all times without being forced to use an appliance.

This anecdotal information is also documented by Bourque (in PERK patients)[1] and by Powers.[2] These studies explored patient motivation by using standard psychometric techniques. The conclusion was that cosmetic advantage is a very small factor in electing RK surgery. Startling to those inexperienced with RK patients, cosmetic reasons for choosing surgery is the dominant factor in only 3% of the cases.

Then why all the concern about whether or not doing or having the procedure is justified? If you accept the erroneous premise that RK is primarily cosmetic surgery, and acknowledge the possibility of serious complications (even if it is less than one in 10,000 cases), then a patient is risking his sight just to improve his appearance. This would not be wise or prudent. A person would have to be vain, foolish, or ill-informed to desire RK. This is not the case, however, since it is easily documented that the surgery restores useful vision and thus is functional.

Radial keratotomy *is definitely* functional surgery and not cosmetic surgery. Patients desire surgery so they can avoid the dangers, risks, inconveniences, and frightening situations that they know will occur when they are caught without their glasses or contact lenses. They are particularly concerned about everyday situations, such as driving the family car, navigating steps and curbs, boating, swimming, and skiing. Walking down city streets, particularly at night, or being able to find an escape route from a burning building also are basic motivations for the surgery. They want to be relieved of their handicapped vision and function in a safe and normal way every minute of every day, and who can blame them?

Opponents of RK have a right, nay, a duty to document the risks, complications, and results of any improperly performed RK. Because they frequently underestimate the patient's natural fear of any surgical procedure, they do not recognize the very cautious approach the patients use in making the decision to have keratotomy surgery. The opponents can call the procedure frivolous, dangerous, and unwise, if that is their interpretation of the scientific facts, but they do not have the right to indict the motives of others, patients or physicians. Likewise, no matter how often or how loudly they repeat it, they do not have the right to create a lie that functional surgery is "cosmetic." It is time for this issue to be resolved. Radial keratotomy is a curative, effective procedure. It is not, and never has been, cosmetic surgery.

References
1. Bourque, L.B., Rubenstein R., Cosand B, et al: "Psychosocial characteristics of candidates for the Prospective Evaluation of Radial Keratotomy (PERK) study," *Arch. Ophthalmol.* 1984; 102: 1187-1192.
2. Powers MK, Meyerowitz BE, Arrowsmith PN, et al: "Psychosocial findings in radial keratotomy patients two years after surgery." *Ophthalmology* 1984; 91: 1193-1198.

Michael R. Deitz, MD
Mission, Kansas

*Reprinted with permission of *The Journal of Refractive Surgery,* from its July-August 1986 issue (Volume 2: Number 4, pages 152-3).